MW01517197

End Result

F I T N E S S

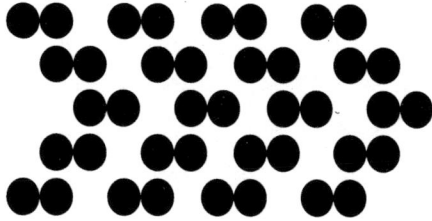

IMPORTANT

The material in this book is for informational purposes only and is not intended as a substitute for the advice and care of your physician. As with all new weight-loss or weight-maintenance regiments, the nutrition program described in this book should be followed only after first consulting with your physician to make sure it is appropriate for your individual circumstances, or if you have questions about your health. Keep in mind that nutrition needs vary from person to person, depending on age, sex, health status, and total diet.

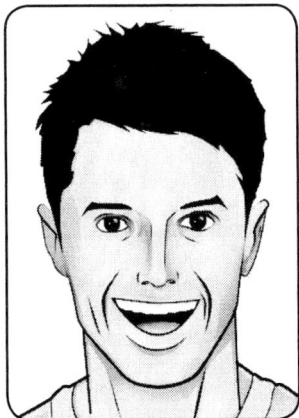

YOUR PERSONAL TRAINER
is with you every step of the way

Author and creator of End Result Fitness, Allan Alguire believes that when it comes to losing weight, getting healthy and improving your life, every day is a new opportunity; a clean slate. With his help, you could improve your life right here, right now and best of all, you can do so in half the time. He knows what it's like having a busy schedule and has designed a proven system that only requires 30 minutes to give you the body you want, the health you need and the life you deserve.

Before Allan created End Result Fitness and shared his motivating advice on TV to inspire thousands of people to become lighter and healthier through proper eating and exercise he was anything but happy with the way he looked and felt. Despite the fact that he was at a very 'healthy' weight by BMI standards, he had far too much body fat and far too little muscle tone. This left him with zero energy, and with an incredibly slow metabolism that would only promote fat gain in the years to come. Allan knows what being unhappy with the way you look and feel is all about. But he took the necessary steps to change his life…….and so can you. He will do everything in his power to help you, to inspire you, and to provide you with as much information as he can to make positive changes in your life. Your job is to take the first step to a better, healthier life for #1…YOU.

While helping thousands of clients just like YOU achieve the end result they want, Allan has come to see that the two biggest issues that you'll face in your journey are not having the willpower to follow a specific nutrition plan and not experiencing fast enough results from your fitness program to stay motivated.

If you're like most people you want to lose weight, feel stronger inside and out and add quality years to your life. Allan will motivate, educate, and support you every step of the way to achieving the end result you want and the life you deserve, regardless of your current fitness level.

When you become a End Result Fitness client/friend you'll benefit from Allan's professional credibility, his understanding of real-life challenges, and his genuine personality. Plus, you'll immediately feel his enthusiasm as well as the energy of the entire End Result Fitness family when you join.

Try End Result Fitness For 90 Days RISK-FREE!
www.EndResultFitness.ca

YOUR End Result

FITNESS

THE FITNESS PLAN
YOU NEED
FOR THE END RESULT
YOU DESERVE!

TABLE OF CONTENTS

INTRODUCTION

Congratulations on taking the first step towards guaranteeing your success with your *NEW Personalized Workout and Nutrition Plan*.

If you're like many people, you've tried program after program after program in the past only to find that you're experiencing far less than stellar results.

After all, if you would have had high level results, you wouldn't be reading this book right now. Instead, you're sitting there thinking, what could I do differently this time around to *ensure* that I don't end up right back in this exact same spot again in a few months time?

The fact of the matter is that the success rate on most diets is incredibly low. You don't need me to tell you that though. All you really need to do is look around you.

You'll find overweight people *everywhere*. In the gym, at the bookstore rummaging through the fat loss and dieting section, or just out and about walking the streets.

It's true, in our world today obesity has become a major issue. And unless people start taking more time out of their day to learn the *right* methods of approaching this problem, it's just going to continue as it is, if not get even worse.

Currently fast food consumption is higher than ever before despite all the research that is being put into various health campaigns running around the nation and all the additional funds being dumped into developing food products that are supposed to be better for our health.

People are still not taking action though to do something about it. But the good news is that you are. At least you're looking for a solution and the even better news is that you've come to the right place.

When you arm yourself with the knowledge, that's when you're going to see nothing but results. No more failed diet attempts, no more frustrating sessions in the gym where you come out *heavier* than you were before, and definitely no more disappointing thoughts that maybe you're just meant to be heavy.

In this book you will discover some very impressive results that the clients I have worked with in the past have obtained. I've helped hundreds of people achieve goals that they previously thought were out of reach; whether they were goals to shed over 100 pounds of fat, goals to add more lean muscle mass so they can prevent fat gain down the road, or goals to get in the absolute best shape possible for an upcoming special event like your wedding day.

Whatever your goals, you can achieve it, if you follow the advice I'm going to present to you.

I have been in the fitness industry for the last 12 years and to say I have 'been there, done that', would be an understatement. I've seen various fitness tricks and techniques come into the mainstream market, and seen just as many *leave* the mainstream market because they just weren't producing the results that people are looking for.

Over the course of time, this also means that I've come to learn exactly what does produce results and get your body in the top shape that you're looking for.

Believe me when I tell you that there are far more gimmicky 'quick-fix's than there are long lasting solutions. If you aren't well-versed in how the body handles exercise and various foods, you likely won't see success because there are just too many misleading programs out there that you might jump onto.

The worst part about this is usually the programs that produce the fewest results promise the most. Thus, faithful followers who *think* they are really doing the right thing are the ones to jump on them but in the process, these incorrect programs just serve to erode their beliefs in themselves and produce long-term disappointment surrounding health and fitness itself.

This just leaves you in a position where you'd rather not think about leading a healthy lifestyle and just accept the status quo.

Never accept the status quo.

If you can dream it, you can achieve it – within reason, of course.

So who's this book for?

This book is for the person who wants to create change. This book is for the person who is ready to challenge their belief systems (and their bodies!) and start seeing results.

This book is for someone who is ready to put in some work.

What you must know is that fat loss doesn't come easy. I really wish I could just wave a wand or offer you some 'magical' pill and instantly make you thin again, but I can't. You know this deep down inside yourself anyway. If there was a successful 'quick-fix' that actually worked to take the weight off and keep it off for good, the obesity problem as we know it would be gone.

But that isn't how it is and weight loss does take some work – and this is why the problem is still present across the nation. Most people just aren't ready to put in the work necessary, so you're already passed the first hurdle.

When we team up together and you start working with End Result Fitness you are going to tap into a wealth of information that you've never experienced before.

Together, we're going to show you all the best methods to get to where you want to be in the shortest amount of time. Basically, every ounce of hard work that you put in will be rewarded with results. No more feeling like you're wasting your time.

Every session counts.

That's our motto and we live by it. We are only going to show you the absolute most effective methods to change your body and help change your life.

So you can be certain in your mind that what you're doing *will* work and you can put those negative self-defeating beliefs behind you.

If this describes you – someone who is ready and prepared to take action, then congratulations again, you're reading the right book.

What you're about to learn will, without a doubt, change the way you look at fitness forever.

So let's not waste any more time and get you the information you've been waiting for.

SECTION 1:
SETTING YOURSELF UP FOR SUCCESS

Before you even dive into your workout programs and get going with the diet, it's important to first take a look at your own personality characteristics as well as your overall lifestyle and the environment that surrounds you to determine whether or not you're in the position to see the best results possible from your efforts.

There are certain factors that should be in place before you get going that will dramatically boost the overall level of results you see, so by making sure these are in place first before you begin, you're going to up the chances that you get started on the right foot.

Many people assume that all they need to do is follow some program and results will come but often it's not quite as straightforward as that.

There is a certain mindset that you should be in that will, without a doubt, help you achieve a much higher level of results and fitness than someone who isn't in the same frame of mind.

By taking the time now to get your environment and mind set correct, you ensure that everything else that follows is going to be 100% effective.

Let's have a look at what you should consider.

CHAPTER 1:
DO YOU HAVE WHAT IT TAKES?

At first thought, you may answer that question with a resounding, 'Of course!' Or, you could be on the opposite end of the spectrum and if you've had a few failed attempts at a fat loss plan in the past, you may answer somewhat hesitantly, not truly knowing if you really are capable of experiencing the results you're after.

Believe it or not, what you think about throughout the day as well as how you react with others will have an immediately DIRECT impact on how you proceed forward.

Your mind is an extremely powerful thing and when it's not 'on' the right page, neither will your success. Your mind essentially controls everything, so it's vital that you get this on track first before moving forward.

The Positive Mindset

First and foremost you must be maintaining a powerful mindset. Far more often than not most of us are constantly saying negative affirmations to ourselves throughout the day which then only serves to degrade our well-being and the efforts we're putting in.

One very good exercise to help make yourself more aware of this is to start catching yourself in these negative self-statements.

Next time you hear yourself say something bad about what you've done, how you're progressing, or anything else related to making these positive behavioural changes in your life, I want you to instantly catch yourself and force yourself to say five positive statements to yourself in place of it.

By doing this, you'll completely flip your mental outlook from a negative one to a positive one, really improving the overall direction that your mind is pointing in.

Start doing this regularly for the next week. Each and every time you have that negative statement, replace it with five positives. It may be hard at first to come up with these positives but do your best and avoid repeating them time and time again. The more variations you can come up with, the better.

And it doesn't necessarily have to be strictly related to your workouts or diet abilities either. These positive statements can be related to other areas of your life where you feel you excel in. The point of all of this is to shift your negative thought patterns towards the positive so that you're less likely to feel incapable and also improve your overall self-esteem in the process.

The second exercise you should be doing is active self-planning. What this refers to is planning out little things that you're going to do each week to improve yourself.

I am a firm believer that we should always be constantly striving for more from ourselves as this is what will help us grow further as individual human beings. The moment you just accept the status quo is the moment you stop growing and usually the moment you stop improving as well.

So the second exercise to do is to get out a pen right now and write down five things you'll do during the coming week that are going to move you one step closer to where you want to be.

Now, this could be finishing this book in its entirety so you're already equipped with the knowledge you need and ready to go, it could be clearing out your pantry of all the processed and junk foods so that you don't end up turning to them down the road when you shouldn't be, or it might be investing in a new pair of running shoes to get ready for the workouts to come.

Whatever it is, you are to find five positive things that you can do to move yourself forward. By doing this you're not only obviously getting ready for success, but you're also going to be giving yourself the sense of accomplishment from doing these tasks.

In our daily lives, we tend to feel a great deal better when we accomplish something that was pre-determined than when it just happens by chance. By doing this pre-planning and then following through, you'll increase something called your self-efficacy, which is essentially how you feel about your ability to complete a task. The higher your self-efficacy, the more success you generally experience.

So there you have two exercises that you should do immediately to get started. Don't wait until you're finished reading the book, you are to do these exercises NOW. There's no better time like the present to get started so do not put this off any longer. Start making improvements to yourself now and you'll be that much closer to seeing positive results in the long run.

The Law Of Reciprocation

Another very important part of the equation to consider is what I like to refer to as the 'law of reciprocation'. What this law is all about is how you treat and influence other people.

Believe it or not, how you treat others comes directly back to how you feel about yourself. Think about it for a second. The last time you gave someone a very well thought out meaningful compliment, how did you feel?

Chances are you felt pretty good. You could tell that this person genuinely appreciated your comment and you made them smile; likely even brightened their day.

And in return, you went away feeling just a little bit better about yourself. After all, you just made someone happier and we as humans tend to feel good about ourselves when that occurs (which is why we also tend to favour people who make us feel better about ourselves and be around them more often than those who don't).

So as you can see, despite the fact that there was nothing in this compliment for you, you actually benefited from it.

This is the exact law that you're going to replicate with the program. What I want you to do is start encouraging *others* to get with the fitness lifestyle and support and encourage them.

Pick out two people that you currently associate with that you feel would be responsive to a little bit of encouragement and make the effort to do so before this exact same time tomorrow.

See what happens.

As you go about doing this, you're going to find that encouraging them also causes you to become more excited about your program and transformation and thus leads to you seeing better results.

Plus, you'll be helping others (again, giving you that 'feel good' feeling that we as humans love so much). You may even find a new workout partner because of it.

Additionally, when you can get those around you in support of a healthy lifestyle, it's going to make it that much easier to maintain one yourself, furthering along the progress that you see.

It's nothing but a win-win situation. The old saying, 'you have to give in order to receive' couldn't apply more to this situation. By giving you really will be receiving in the end.

So those are the first two main things that you absolutely must remember when it comes to your mindset. How you think and what you do with your thoughts are two extremely powerful components that you absolutely must be paying attention to.

Let's look at the third.

Workout With a Group

One of the best ways to set yourself up for success is to workout with a group rather than alone. When you come to workout with End Result Fitness, very often group sessions will be utilized so that you get that added motivational support from the other person or people in the group and form lifelong friendships in the process.

When working out in a group you're going to find that the entire feeling of energy is much higher and the overall workout is that much more enjoyable.

Not enough can be said about the positive experience of working out with one or two other people over that of going about it alone.

Strive For Progress Over Perfection

Perfection. It's a word that most of us feel slightly anxious about whenever we see or hear it because for many, it immediately brings thoughts of our own shortcomings to mind.

Or instead we may think about how far away from perfection we currently are. But yet, many of us, when we set out on a diet or workout program strive for just that. Rather than focusing on all the vast improvements we are making and how far we've come in a short period of time, we instead look at all the things we still have yet to accomplish and how far away we are from our ideal.

This needs to stop.

When you strive for perfection you will always be setting yourself up for disappointment because as you very likely already know, perfection just can't be reached.

In fact, if you were to envision someone who you consider 'perfect' – this ideal image you have and likely what you are in fact trying to obtain and ask them whether or not they felt perfect, you'd get a far different answer.

Each and every one of us sees shortcomings in ourselves. Some obviously see more than others. But usually, this has more to do with our own self-beliefs and self-confidence than actual physical shortcomings that are actually present.

When you can focus on the good things about yourself and spend less energy thinking about the bad, you'll actually feel much closer to the ideal than you currently do.

What you must be doing though as you work through this process of reaching your ideal body and even once you have is focusing on *progression* not *perfection*.

The two are vastly different and will impact your thoughts in entirely different manners. When you focus on progress, you see success.

When you focus on perfection, you'll see failure.

See the difference?

Now, which do you think is going to be best for boosting your self-esteem and your belief that your program is actually working? Obviously progression is. Progression you can see. You can really see those day to day improvements that are moving you forward towards your goal.

Perfect, now that's an end point – something that you just hope to reach. But, reality is that you'll never reach it as it's usually impossible to be absolutely perfect. Even when you obtain what you thought was 'perfect', you now realize that there's something else that's even better that now represents a new perfect for you.

The point is that chasing perfection is a futile effort. If you want to actually move forward, chase after day to day improvements that you can recognize. Inch by inch you'll get there. Step by step you'll see positive changes. And eventually, after it all adds up together, you will reach the ideal you have set out for yourself.

No, you may not be perfect, but you'll be happy and that at the end of the day is what counts.

This isn't to say that you should strive for less than what you think is actually possible. That's not the point at all. You should set your sights on a goal that is really going to challenge you to become that much better than you currently are but with this goal, you must ensure that it's realistic.

If your goal isn't realistic, you're going to be disappointed so you might as well get this right at the start. Failing to set appropriate smart goals is going to come back to haunt you later on.

Once you have your goals set, then the other factors that will need to be in place for success to occur include determination, perseverance, commitment, and then the proven results plan that you'll get from working with End Result Fitness.

Want to see just what the combination of these factors can produce? Take a look at some of the recent client testimonials. All of these people focused on progression and not perfection and then had all four factors working in their favour.

Laurie:
I decided to try End Result Fitness because I wanted to look and feel my personal best on my wedding day.

I then continued with End Result Fitness to ensure I stayed lean, toned and strong throughout my first and second pregnancy.

I was able to lose my pregnancy weight - fast! I now look and feel the same way I did on my wedding day.

STAYED LEAN, TONED AND STRONG THROUGHOUT HER PREGNANCY

Carl:
I decided to try End Result Fitness because I was border line obese and was developing muscle imbalances which was worsening my posture problems.

I was able to lose over 50 lbs of body fat and correct all my muscle imbalances.

I'm now my ideal weight, have better posture and feel confident in my own body.

Before
After
LOST 50 LBS OF BODY FAT

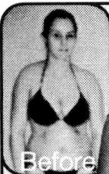

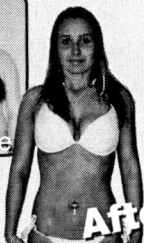

Melanie:

I used to weigh 130lbs and had a body fat percentage of 29.5%. By BMI standards I was my "ideal weight" but when wearing a bikini I felt obese! I now love the way I look and feel in my bikini now that I'm 114lbs with 17% body fat. I really thank End Result Fitness for all the support in helping me renew my confidence and love for life!

Before

After

LOST 12.5% BODY FAT

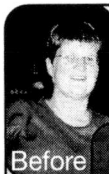

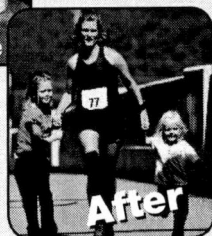

Gillian:

I was over 250 pounds and all the extra body fat was wreaking havoc on my circulation, causing me numbness and pain. I knew that this was a sign of type II diabetes. I wanted to lose the weight for me and my daughters! End Result Fitness introduced me to resistance training and proper nutrition. Allan made my workouts safe, effective and fun. I now do 3 full marathons a year along with numerous other races with my daughters. My quality of life has improved tremendously.

Before

After

LOST OVER 125 LBS OF BODY FAT FOR HER DAUGHTERS

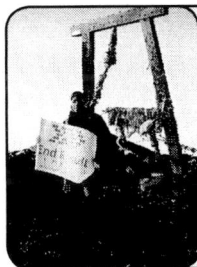

Craig:

I was able to lean out and tone up my entire body and build the strength needed to climb Mt. Fuji while following the End Result Fitness system. I love that I only had to workout 3 times per week for ONLY 30 minutes to see results fast. With my busy schedule, this was very convenient. Thanks Allan for motivating, educating and supporting me every step of the way.

BUILT THE STRENGTH TO CLIMB MOUNT FUJI

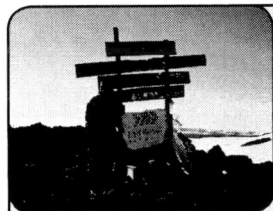

Debbie:

From the first time I saw Mount Kilimanjaro I wanted to make the trek to the summit. I finally decided to stop procrastination and contacted Allan to get me into shape. His expertise, and tremendous positive attitude was exactly what I needed to meet the challenge. Thanks Allan for all the personalized programs and nutrition plans that I needed to meet the challenge and succeed.

CLIMBED MOUNT KILIMANJARO AND SUCCEEDED

So now you can clearly see just how strongly this combination is. When you get the mind working with the body and then also have a powerful workout and diet plan, success will seem easy.

Now let's move on to our next topic, that of taking pre-transformation statistics.

CHAPTER 2:
TAKING YOUR PRE-TRANSFORMATION STATS

Before you get going with your new workout plan designed to completely change how you look, it's vital that you get that starting point reference.

How will you know how far you've come if you never have anything to look back from? You've seen them many times before – those before and after pictures that grace the pages of magazines or websites.

You even saw a few of the clients that have worked with End Result Fitness and achieved great success only to carry on setting new goals and move up to an even greater level of fitness than they ever imagined possible. Now you are about to become your own before and after success story.

By taking your 'before' pictures and measurements at this point, you will have that to use to propel you forwards. Sometimes weight loss can seem like a slow process. There may be weeks where you work hard yet don't notice a very large impact in the image staring back at you in the mirror.

Usually, this leads to much disappointment among those who are putting in the effort and who are working very hard to get to where they want to be.

But when you have sheer statistics that you can use, then it's far easier to see numerical progress when sometimes the eye isn't seeing the progress it would like.

For example, let's say one week goes by and you don't drop a pound on the scale. But since muscle is far more dense tissue you may have actually noticed your waist measurement went down an inch despite this lack of adjustment on the scale number reading back to you.

Would you have noticed this inch reduction without measurements? Likely not – unless you have very well trained eyes. This is why taking some starting measurements is vital.

Likewise, when motivation levels are low and you feel as though you'll never reach your *end result*, it can really help to look at pictures of yourself when you first started. Usually this will put it back into your direct reference just how far you have really come and how close you are getting to your *end result*.

If you've lost a good 20-30 pounds, make no mistake about it, you're going to look quite a bit different. By looking back over that difference, it can really serve to motivate you to keep going as you then can clearly see just how much of a difference your effort is really making.

So what should you do to get these statistics?

First comes the photo. This is going to be a picture of yourself, preferably in as little clothing as possible (you do want to see your current shape here) representing where you stand right now.

Label this your 'GOOD BYE PHOTO'. As in you will never look like this again because positive changes are headed your way.

Once you have this picture (and do make sure it is clear so you can make out all the little lines and folds you may happen to have) of the front profile, the back profile, as well as the side profile then you also need to get your stats.

For this, you're going to take your girth measurement as well as any measurements of other body parts that you're trying to work on. For instance, if you want to slim your legs, take a measurement of the circumference of your thigh.

If you want to tone your arms, take the measurement of your arms instead. Wherever you want to make some changes be sure that you have a corresponding measurement to go along with it.

Then, the next thing you'll need is your body weight measurements. You can get this by standing on a scale (preferably in the morning before you've eaten or drank anything but after going to the washroom) as well as your BMI.

To get your BMI, use this equation:

$$BMI = \text{weight in kilograms} / (\text{height in meters})^2$$

Now that you have those two readings, you'll need your body fat. Body fat is by far the most important tracking method to use because this essentially tells you exactly what is going on with your body composition.

Body composition is something that's incredibly important to know because it can denote whether you are what's called 'skinny fat'.

Let me explain skinny fat for a second. Basically skinny fat is where you are actually relatively quite thin – you may even be at a relatively low body weight however you have a very high overall level of body fat with little to no muscle definition.

So what you get as a result is a thin person who looks and feels flabby. Not very attractive – is it? Being skinny fat is a dangerous position to be in because not only are you still at many health risks due to your higher overall body fat percentage but you also lack the muscle mass that's going to keep your metabolism running high.

In the name of fat loss, having a high metabolism is going to be absolutely critical to success. You wouldn't want to go without it.

Whenever someone sets the goal to be 'skinny', you must define this. You can be 'skinny' and still not look very good in a bathing suit at all if you have excess fat on your body. Instead, you want to be firm and toned – thin yet fit. That creates a much better picture.

Ideally, you want to notice your body fat percentage going down while your lean mass weight stays constant. This is a clear indication that you are losing body fat and not losing muscle mass.

If you instead notice that the scale weight is dropping but your total body fat percentage is staying the same or possibly even increasing, then 'Houston, we have a problem'. This measurement is vital so be sure you get it done.

The best bet will be to get a body fat test done using skin callipers which will measure various areas of the body for the skin-fold thickness. Usually places to be measured include your abdomen, the underarm, the area by your shoulder blades, the chest, as well as the thigh and the calf. Whomever you have testing your body fat will know the exact location to use so trust their judgement while having it done.

Moving forward, next you need to figure out your BMR (basal metabolic rate). What your BMR is going to measure is how many calories you are burning up on a daily basis just to stay alive.

Essentially if you did nothing but lay in bed all day long without moving a muscle, this is how many calories you would burn. Those who have faster metabolisms usually have an easier time maintaining their body weight and losing fat when on a diet while those who have slower metabolisms have a harder time doing so.

Lean muscle tissue is one of the biggest predictors of what your basal metabolic rate will be, so once again, protecting it is in your best interest. It's also the tissue that's going to really up your overall calorie burn.

For example, one pound of muscle mass will burn off about 50-75 calories per day while one pound of fat will burn off a measly 2 calories.

Imagine how much of a difference adding 10 pounds of lean muscle tissue to your body would make! You could increase your metabolic rate by up to 750 calories each and every day! This means you could eat that much more food without worrying about fat gain or you could eat as you are and lose up to 1 to 1.5 pounds of fat more each week. No additional exercise required!

Now there are two ways to go about getting your BMR. There's the scientific-formula route for those who are math inclined and then there's the 'good approximation' method for those who aren't.

Let's start with the science.

One of the most accurate predictors of the basal metabolic rate is the Harris Benedict Equation which is:

Women: BMR = 655 + (4.35 X weight in pounds) + (4.7 X height in inches) – (4.7 X age in years)

Men: BMR = 66 + (6.23 X weight in pounds) + (12.7 X height in inches) – (6.8 X age in years)

This will give you a fairly good estimation of your general daily calorie requirements to sustain life.

Now, if you prefer the simpler method, simply take your current body weight (in pounds) and multiply by a factor of 10 for women and 11 for men.

Usually you'll find that this gives you a number that is quite close to that of the formulas provided, so it also serves as a good starting point to follow.

Note though that neither of these equations are going to be ideal for someone who is either very muscular and lean or someone who is very high in overall body fat.

These individuals will usually have swayed results by these equations because they have so much of one type of body mass that either burns so few calories per day (fat) or burns so many calories per day (muscle mass).

In that situation, then you need the lean body mass calculator.

For this one you have:

BMR = 370 + (21.6 X lean mass in kg's)

This equation is the same for both males and females so you don't have to worry about adjusting it based on your gender.

If you want to use this equation, think back to where you figured out your total body fat percentage and then use that to work backwards to determine your lean mass in kg's.

Let's say you arrived at 22% body fat, you would take your body weight (let's use 150 pounds for example's sake) and multiple that by 0.22 (percent body fat).

This gives you 33 pounds of fat total. So now you know you have 33 pounds of body fat on your frame. You then take 150 minus those 33 pounds to get 117 pounds of lean body mass total. Divide by 2.2 to get this in kg's and you're now ready to use that equation.

As you go about the process of fat loss it's going to be important to continually keep checking this equation because as you lose weight, you're going to find that it goes down slightly.

Since your BMR accounts for a good part of determining how much food you need to eat on a daily basis (which you'll learn about later on), it's a vital statistic that you must be accurate on.

Finally, the last stat that you'll need to do is a fitness test. This test should assess both your strength, cardiovascular, and recovery levels and can be done quickly and effectively at End Result Fitness.

You'll find that you're doing these tests on an ongoing basis as you go about your training with us as well, as it's going to be what makes us certain that you're progressing forwards and allows us to determine the best changes to make with your program.

The recordings that you get back from this test will also be important to determine how far you've come in terms of your overall fitness level as you progress through the program.

So there you have it – all the main tests to do *before* you dive into your program. By taking the time now to do them, you will have a very good reference for tracking your progress and making sure that you are moving forward in the manner you would like to.

Now let's get into chapter three and talk a little bit about overcoming hurdles and being prepared. This is important!

CHAPTER 3:
PREPARING YOURSELF TO OVERCOME HURDLES

Now that we've discussed making sure that you're in the proper mindset to get yourself on track to seeing a high level of results, it's time to start thinking about any obstacles that could be headed your way at this point and what you can do to overcome them.

There's no question that there will come a point in your program where something comes up and really throws you off course.

Whether it's a work meeting that has gone late and is forcing you to skip out on your workout session or it's an injury that has taken place that is making you take some time off while you heal, things will come up and you must deal with them.

Often those that aren't as prepared to handle these hurdles are going to be far more likely to just throw in the towel at that point and really let this hurdle impact their progress in the long run.

That's why having a back-up plan is absolutely vital. Without it, you're just going to struggle along the program, constantly feeling as though you're just barely hanging on.

One exercise that you should begin immediately is to take the time to think of ten hurdles that you may encounter in your own life.

And remember, these don't necessarily have to be attendance related hurdles. They could be a bad mindset, negative comments given by others, a lack of proper food in the house when you need it, or anything else that you know in your life could come up.

Each and every one of us battles different hurdles so it's vital that you realize what's going to come into play in your own situation.

So right now, take the time to do this. List out ten hurdles that you could foresee possibly having to face.

Got them?

Now that these are down, what I want you to do is list out three potential solutions to overcome these hurdle. These solutions could be alternatives to use in the case this problem comes up, ways that you'll talk yourself around the hurdle so you'll get back on your plan, or perhaps someone you'll consult to help get you through it.

You know your own life best so it's time to put this knowledge into action. Take the time to figure out what you'll have to do to get past this hurdle now so that when it does come up, you're ready to go with your action-plan.

Once again, failing to have a plan is planning to fail so never go without. If there's one thing that you can do that will guarantee that you see success with transforming your body, having a plan is it.

Okay, now what you must do is read over these on a daily basis. You want to really get them ingrained in your mind so that should that hurdle creep up, you have an automatic tendency to rely on your back-up plan to get you through it. You want this process to be automatic.

Hurdle ====> Back-up plan.

The more automatic you make it, the stronger the chance you will see success.

Great, so now you're primed and ready to go and nothing is going to get in your way.

Before we move on to our next topic, let's give you ten success tips that you should be following.

Success Tip #1:
Get Groceries Every Sunday

One of the most helpful tips that you can ever make use of if you want to succeed with fat loss is to make sure that you do as much of your grocery shopping as you can over the weekend.

As soon as the weekday's hit you're going to find that you're incredibly busy and grocery shopping often falls off your to-do list. When this happens, that's when you're also far more likely to turn to quick-fix dinner solutions that are likely to be anything but healthy.

If you can get as many of the staples that you need in your fridge, cupboard, and freezer then you'll feel less pressure throughout the week to go about getting what you require.

Remember too that you can precook many of your meals and place them in the freezer over the weekend as well. This little trick can save hours of cooking time over the course of the week so it's definitely one to make use of. If you're going to spend time cooking you might as well cook larger batches so it makes things easier on you during the week.

Do as much as you can to get ready for your weekday meals on the weekend and you'll have that much of a better chance of sticking with your diet plan.

Success Tip #2:
Envision Your Success For Five Minutes Per Day

Second, the next thing that you must do if you want to realize success is take some time out to envision yourself seeing success for five minutes out of the day. Sit there and really picture what it's going to be like when you reach your goal.

Try to really imagine what you're going to feel like, look like, how you'll act, the things you'll say, and the reaction you'll get from others around you.

Basically, you want to 'live the dream'. By doing this, it helps you paint the picture of what it is you're going for here and helps you really put yourself in the shoes of what it will be like when you achieve your goals.

By doing this, you're going to find that it also deepens your 'hunger' for success so much that you're far more devoted to carrying out your program plan than you were before.

If we never really get a 'taste' for success, it's hard to picture ourselves there. And in real life, you can't magically make yourself your goal weight for just a day or two, but by imagining it long enough, you can get a pretty close feel for where you'll be in a few months time with some good, hard work.

Some people also find that talking with other people about their goals and their progression is a great way to increase a higher thirst for success. In addition to increasing your own desire to reach your goals, this may spark interest in whomever you're talking to as well, and then you can easily refer them back to End Result Fitness so they too can realize their true potential.

Remember, when you are working together with friends and family at improving your health and fitness level, the results tend to be that much more dramatic.

Success Tip #3:
Stay In The Present, Not The Past

Third, another important success tip that you must remember is to always stay in the present. Don't ever let yourself ruminate in the past and your previous mistakes. Look to the future and concentrate on the present.

Remember, you can't change the past and by dwelling on it, all you do is hinder your progression into the future. If you want to keep moving forward, that's where your attention needs to be.

We as humans have a strong tendency to create our present situation so to speak with where our mind is at and by constantly being mentally present in the past, the past is what will become of your future.

So the moral of this story is that you must leave the past in the past. Don't keep thinking about it otherwise it will become, right before your eyes, your future.

Success Tip #4:
Schedule Those Workouts

Fourth, be sure to take the time each week to also schedule your workouts. Just like you're scheduling your meal planning, you also must be scheduling in your gym sessions. If you do this, you'll be that much less likely to skip out on them.

Don't leave those workouts up to chance. Put them into your day planner like you would a doctor's appointment and you will be there – on time.

This is another advantage to working with End Result Fitness – by making the commitment to your sessions where you know we'll be waiting to work with you, you'll feel that much more compelled to show up, thus really boosting your overall level of progress.

Success Tip #5:
Remember The 90/10 Rule

Success tip #5 has to do with making sure that you keep the 'big picture' in mind. How many times have you swayed from your diet and then felt incredibly guilty because of it? Too many times to count?

If so, don't feel bad, you certainly aren't alone.

Many people get stuck in the notion that they must follow their diet to the letter and if they don't, they've done horribly wrong.

While you definitely should be putting in the effort to eat properly and maintain the plan you have set for yourself, remember that every diet should have some room for fun. If it doesn't, it's not that well thought out of a plan.

Ideally, you should be trying to follow the 90/10 rule. What this rule states is that 90% of the time you're 'on', while 10% of the time you're having some fun.

If you want some ice cream – have it.

Want to make it chicken wings? – It's fair game.

Whatever you're craving, give in. Later on we'll go over some smart strategies that you can use to actually ensure that you get these treats in there without seeing weight gain because of it.

Quite in fact, when you follow the diet advice that we recommend here when you work with us, these treats will actually help you lose body fat *faster*.

Yes, you read that right. We've developed tricks that actually cause the body to go into fat loss overdrive when you implement cheat meals properly and you'll learn them all yourself.

This means you'll never have to feel deprived again while following a plan. Instead you'll feel satisfied, full of energy, and healthy, all while seeing the fat loss that you're after.

Success Tip #6:
Keep Yourself Honest

Moving on to success tip #6, this one is all about honesty. When you're on your body transformation plan, you must ensure that you're keeping yourself honest. Far too many people will let themselves slip but then not acknowledge they are doing so.

It's almost like they go into some form of self-denial where they cheat on their plans or skip workouts but then look for something else to blame for why they are not seeing results.

If you're going to skip a workout, admit to it. You don't have to beat yourself up for it, but be honest about it and why you're doing it. This is a must if you're going to progress forward and find solutions to why you are skipping the workouts like you are.

If you aren't doing these things as you should, it's imperative that you're honest and work towards a solution. If you keep yourself in denial results will never come and worst of all, you'll have absolutely no reason why they are not.

Don't repress your mistakes. Bring them out to conscious awareness and then attack them with solutions.

Success Tip #7:
Don't Be Afraid To Ask For Help

Another key thing that you must be sure to remember is that you never have to go about this journey alone. Far too many people don't take the effort to seek out the help they need when they need it.

Whether you need a good personal trainer to get you through the rough patches of your weight loss or you require some specific nutritional advice for a certain situation you're battling, you can get the help you need and overcome whatever it is you're dealing with.

At End Result Fitness we cater to every problem you have so you never have to be shy about explaining your situation. We will figure out the solution that will work for you – and then work with you to put that solution into place.

In other situations, it may be a counsellor that you require. Perhaps you have some very strong emotional issues you're dealing with from the past or the current situation in your life and this is causing you to turn to food for comfort six nights out of the week. Something like this is likely not going to be solved by starting up on a diet and will need some good counselling support to talk you through it.

Again, don't let yourself pass it by. Get the help you need so you can get the *end result* you want. It's far simpler this way if you just open up and let others in.

Success Tip #8:
Get Up Earlier

Now, back to behavioural changes, another quick tip that you may want to consider applying to your life is to aim to get up earlier each and every day. Those that start their day off early typically find they get far more accomplished throughout that day thus they make greater gains towards their goals.

If you've ever slept in until noon, woken up and realized that you only have half the day left, you've likely experienced this phenomenon at work.

This also doesn't take into account the fact that most people are also more productive in the early morning as their mind is just thinking more clearly thus they're far able to get more work done.

Whether it's fitness or other tasks you're performing, early morning is often a very good time if you're looking for results.

As an added benefit, those who get into the habit of doing their workouts first thing in the morning are far more likely to stick with them since there is a lower chance that something else will crowd them out.

Success Tip #9:
Make Time For You

In today's busy world, one thing that many people find is that they never make enough time for them. You're tending to other people's needs 15 hours out of the day and by the time you finish up, you're too exhausted to do anything for yourself.

There's no question that making the time to do your workouts will help out in that regard, but even more importantly you should also be taking the time to spend at least one <u>hour</u> each week doing something that you truly, and 100% enjoy.

By doing this you'll really help to lower your overall levels of stress and 'recharge' your batteries. If you never get the chance to do this you're going to be very burned out quickly and this will really hinder the progress you make not only in terms of your fitness program and body fat loss but in terms of other areas of your life as well.

When we feel good we perform better at everything – work, school, and relationships so it's important that you do make the time for you. Do whatever it takes to free up just a single hour.

This reminds me of a great quote by Deion Snaders:

When You look good, you feel good. When You feel good, you play good and when You play good, the PAY is good!

Don't ever underestimate the influence getting in great shape can have on your overall life. The fact of the matter is that how you feel about your body is a direct influence over how confident you are.

And, how confident you are has a direct influence over how you approach your job, how you approach your finances, and how you approach others who come in and out of your life.

When you feel great, you'll be more confident and show it. This could quite in fact lead to things like a sparked new relationship or a job promotion.

This isn't to say if you lose weight you'll become rich – you have to put in the hard work to do so but never discount the power of confident. Weight loss will bring you confidence.

Success Tip #10:
Realize Your Successes

Finally, the last success tip that you must be following is to do just that – realize your success.

Don't ever underestimate your capabilities and the small things that you accomplish on a day to day basis. Don't undervalue yourself or talk down about what you have done.

Be proud of your accomplishments and remind yourself of them daily.

This doesn't necessarily mean you have to go off building an ego higher than Mount Everest but the vast majority of people never even take the time to realize their true value and what they are able to do very effectively in their own life.

When you start to value yourself more as a person like this you'll automatically invest more energy into yourself to grow and develop that more success will just come naturally.

There's that old saying out there that 'some people tend to have all the luck'. If you believe this, you may need a slight attitude adjustment.

While there is no question that certain people do tend to just luck out in life, for the most part, people really do create their own luck. They do this by seeking out opportunities that other people may otherwise not notice and then acting on these opportunities at the right time.

But, they are also very self-confident about their own abilities as they strongly value themselves and have realized their past successes so this self-confidence gives them the chance to act while others may have just passed it by.

Start being more receptive to your own successes – no matter how small – and you may just find that luck starts finding you a little more often.

Once again, this applies not only to fitness and fat loss, but to all other areas of your life as well.

So there you have ten quick success tips that you should be following. If you are ready to get on the path to results, be sure that you don't overlook any of them.

Now let's carry on and begin to look at what's required for the 'fat loss environment'.

CHAPTER 4:
THE FAT LOSS ENVIRONMENT

Having the right diet program in check and workout plan ready are definitely two of the most critical aspects in order to achieve success with your goals. But, along with having both of those in place, another vital element that should be considered is what I like to call, 'the fat loss environment'.

What's the 'fat loss environment'? Well, this is essentially everything that surrounds you as you go about the program. If you don't have a good environment to carry out the program with, your chances of having setbacks are going to be much higher which is just going to make it feel like you're pulling teeth to stick with the program.

But, when you can get your environment working for you, then you're off to the races. Fat loss will never seem easier since then things just fall into place.

What should you do to ensure that you're creating that perfect fat loss environment for yourself? Let's have a look at a few of the vital things that should be in place.

Support System

Right off the top, the number one thing that you want to ensure you have in place is a good support system. When those people that are around you on a daily basis are in full support of all the efforts you're putting in to reach your goals, this is going to make things far easier on yourself.

Ideally it would be great if your partner (if you are living with someone) was on the program with you as well. When two people are constantly cooking healthy meals and are doing workouts together, the chances of success greatly improve.

Try and refer your friends and family who are taking an interest in your activities to End Result Fitness. We love working in groups with our clients and this will without a doubt help create a more positive environment for you.

If you're constantly preparing separate dishes from the people you live with this will really wear on you in time so if you have others around you who don't mind maintaining a similar diet, not only will cooking be easier, but you won't feel as though you're really being a nuisance to others always eating your own foods.

Not that you can overcome this if it is the case – plenty of people do – but remember, we're trying to set up the ideal environment here so that you see nothing but results.

Easy Access To Your Workout

Second, in your fat loss environment you also want to ensure that you have easy access to your workout facilities. Many of you are going to get into training right in the comfort of your own home, which is a great idea. If you were to pair a few workouts at home with a few workouts with End Result Fitness, you would be right on top of the game for everything you need to see a complete body transformation. There are plenty of exercises to perform in your living room or basement with minimal equipment, so never let having to have a gym membership be a barrier to your success.

If you do choose to workout at a gym as well, then be sure it's readily available. Don't select a place to workout that takes an hour to get to as that will just add unnecessary driving time to your day and you'll be that much less likely to do it. Most people have a hard enough time fitting in the workout itself, let alone fitting in all that time spent travelling.

Fully Stocked Kitchen

Next, also be sure that you have a kitchen that is all stocked up ready to go and is 100% conducive to supporting your diet. Do an all-cupboard clean out at one point when you get a chance where you remove any foods that could potentially set you back.

If the temptation is there, cravings may be satisfied. Be sure to get rid of anything in your fridge or freezer that would not be added to your diet plan as well as having these items in the house is going to make it that much more likely that you sway from your eating strategy.

If you want to keep one or two treats around for when you do actually have a planned 'cheat' meal that's fine, but limit the amount of variety you stock. The more variety, the more you'll want to 'taste' everything.

Even better is if you choose to only purchase those foods the day you are scheduled to have that cheat. This is the top solution to sticking with your plan.

Most people when a craving strikes, will not actually drive out to the grocery or convenience store to pick up whatever it is they're craving. By getting these foods out now, you'll make you life ten times easier in the long run.

Positive Self-Reminders

You should try and create a few positive self-reminders that you can place all around the house to remind you of why you are working towards these goals.

These could be small sticky notes that are placed on the fridge stating why you're eating healthy and reminding you not to snack when you shouldn't or a sheet of paper on your nightstand that you read every morning and every night outlining your goals and how much it means to you that you reach them.

You may also want to get a few picture reminders – which would be a few images of the 'goal body' that you hope to obtain. Looking at these regularly, especially before you head out for a workout is one of the best ways to motivate yourself to push as hard as you possibly can.

Try and figure out which type of reminders are going to work best for you personally. Everyone is slightly different so this is a very personal thing that you must assess and learn from. Some may work better than others so as you progress through the program, you'll see what techniques really work for you to best keep you on track.

Remember, the best way to stay motivated is to prevent losing motivation in the first place. These will help you do just that.

Low Levels Of Negativity

Along with the support system, you must also try and reduce any and all negativity that you may encounter. You should aim to limit contact with any people who are currently in your life who are not supportive of your goals and who are making comments that make you feel less worthy or tend to cause you to fall off the plan.

Now, this is where things can get a little tricky. Obviously there are some people who you just can't eliminate from your life, whether you like it or not, they will be around you. This would be people such as directly related family or a co-worker. In this scenario, your best bet is to talk to the person and discuss how you feel.

Usually if you tell them your reasons for making these positive life changes they will watch what they say around you and they may come to understand just how important your goals are to you.

If they still will not change their ways and continue on with their negativity directed towards you, then you're just going to have to try and avoid them as much as possible. Since you can't avoid them entirely just always remember that they likely have some underlying motive for speaking the way they do to you and more often than not it's about them, not you.

Also keep in mind that very often we perceive people to be more negative than they really are and our defence mechanism immediately goes up.

No one can make you feel inferior about yourself other than you, so if you simply don't give their comments that power over you, you shouldn't have too hard of a time overseeing it.

Of course this is easier said than done at first, but the more you progress along with the program and the more confident you get in your abilities to stick with it, the easier it will be to block out any negativity that comes your way and just let it brush right off of you.

A Mentor

Finally, the last thing that you need in your fat loss environment is a mentor. A mentor is someone who you not only look up to, but someone who you often want to be much like.

This person may not just be someone with a 'hot body' that you wish to obtain, but usually it's someone who also has personality traits that you envy and just a whole persona that you find very appealing.

This is someone who inspires you and keeps you motivated. Someone who you find makes you feel more focused on becoming a better version of yourself. Finally, it's someone who you can hopefully talk to.

In some cases a mentor may not be available to you (if this person is someone you've never met in real life) but then this makes them more of an idol than a mentor.

Your mentor ideally needs to be someone who you are able to reach out to when you're struggling for advice and support. If you can contact them on a daily or semi-weekly basis, all the better.

Many people use personal trainers as mentors since they are, or should be, living out the healthy lifestyle that you hope to obtain. They are also able to give you advice when you need it and serve to motivate you when you're feeling down.

Whomever you choose to use as your mentor, select them carefully because when you do choose the right person, this can have a very large influence over the success you see.

It is possible to also have more than one mentor, as different people may encompass different character traits that you wish to build into your own life, so consider that factor as well.

So there you have all the main things that are going to make-up your fat loss environment. By making sure that you get these on track you will step forth into your program with a greater chance of success.

Most of these are controllable factors, so there should be no reason why you can't at least make some improvements to the current situation you're living in today.

Now let's move forward and talk a bit about goal setting. This too is essential for success, so get ready to do a bit of note taking and planning.

CHAPTER 5:
HOW TO SET SMART GOALS

The one thing almost everyone will naturally do to some extent when getting started on a body transformation challenge is setting some goals. You have to have some desire to get started on a program and this desire is going to stem from whatever your selected goal is.

The problem though is that some people don't necessarily set 'smart' goals. They have goals, make no mistake about that, but their goals are not formulated for success.

So right off the bat what you want to do is make sure that your goals are in check and where they need to be.

Let's talk about what makes up SMART goal setting.

'S' The S in smart goal setting comes from *specific*. This means that whatever your goal is, you must be specific. Don't say that you want to lose weight. That doesn't tell you anything. You could see the scale go down a pound and hooray! – you've just reached your goal.

Not quite. Give details. How much fat do you want to lose? 10 pounds? 20 pounds? Or, do you want to drop 2 dress sizes? The more specific you can be, the better chance you have of reaching your *end result*.

This also gives you a much higher satisfaction level upon reaching your goal since you know, without a question of a doubt, that yes, it's mission accomplished.

'M' The M in smart goal setting comes from *measurable*. What good is a goal if you can't measure it? True, there are some goals – increased energy, improved mood, and so on that you can't really measure statistically but usually these are goals that will accompany other stated goals.

Measurable goals would include things such as body fat levels, the amount of weight you're able to lift, how fast you can run a mile, what your blood pressure reading is, what your cholesterol measurements are, and so on. These are all things that are easily tracked so that you can clearly see how you're progressing along.

This also serves as a great motivational tool since you can spot day to day progress. When you can't really define and measure something, it's much easier to feel as though you're not moving forward.

'A' The A is for *attainable*. This means that given your current situation and lifestyle, you can attain the goal you have set for yourself. For example, let's say you set the goal that you want to run a marathon, but you work 60 hours a week, have two kids, and are the president of your daughter's soccer committee. Do you really think you'll be able to devote a good 20+ hours per week to your training? Likely not – and this is what it takes to reach that type of goal.

It's important that you only select goals that you could reach. If you don't, you're just going to wind up frustrated and eventually give up.

When you consult with us at End Result Fitness we will help ensure that the goals that you are setting are attainable and you'll likely be able to set more lofty goals because of the fact that you'll have us right by your side working with you.

'R' Moving on to R, this stands for *realistic*. Very similar to attainable, realistic stands for goals that are something that you could realistically achieve with enough work put in.

For example, if you're 150 pounds and want to drop 10 pounds of body fat in 6 weeks, that is realistic. If you're 150 pounds and want to drop 10 pounds of body fat in 2 weeks, that likely is not.

Realistic goals help ensure that you do actually have a chance of seeing success. Some people do make the big mistake of setting goals that simply aren't realistic given their situation and this only erodes their self-confidence level when they don't achieve it.

Often they do absolutely nothing wrong with their workout or diet, it's just that they simply did not have a realistic goal they were striving for.

Again, this is something we'll be helping you out with if you're uncertain.

'T'. Finally, the T stands for *timeline*. This is potentially the most important of all the factors because it is what will keep you accountable. Having a specific end date of when you hope to achieve your goal is vital since then you won't be as tempted to slack off when you shouldn't.

We as humans have a very strong tendency to put off tasks that don't have a due date, especially those that we may not find particularly appealing, so this means that if you let your goal date float around, you'll likely never reach that end point.

Instead, give yourself a deadline. You either make it or you don't. If you find you've skipped a few sessions and that deadline is rapidly approaching, this may be enough to kick your butt into gear and get you moving on again towards your goals.

Obviously you also have to ensure that this timeline is realistic. That goes without saying. If you set a timeline that isn't right for the goal you want to achieve that essentially makes the goal unrealistic in itself.

So there you have all the main components of setting SMART goals. Have a look over your current goals. How do they measure up? Could you make a few adjustments?

Remember, you should also be setting some short-term goals as well as some long-term goals. This is what will keep you moving along on your path as we suggested before.

Every time you reach one of your short-term goals you'll feel just a little bit better about yourself and this will help to motivate you further to continue to strive for the next.

If you only have your long-term goal that you're working towards, it's going to be a long time coming before you feel any sense of accomplishment and this can easily cause you to drop off the wagon.

Short term goals should be achieved every 2-4 weeks while long term goals can span across 3-6 months. If you follow this timeline, you'll be right on track.

So right now what you are to do is get out a pen and paper and write down all the goals that you have for yourself, both short and long term. Make sure they qualify as SMART goals and be sure to also write down your reasons why you decided to choose these goals. Why are they important to you?

As you do this, please make sure that you're putting it into your *success journal*. This is the place where you want to track as much as possible so you always have it to refer back to.

All of these tools and resources that we provide to you on a regular basis are designed with your *end result* in mind so take care to utilize them regularly.

Your reasons are the primary things that will serve to keep you motivated so don't skip over that step. Without a reason, a goal is nothing more than a statement on blank paper.

Now remember, you should also be re-evaluating these goals regularly as you progress throughout your training. As you get closer and closer to reaching the various goals you set, you may also find that some of your goals change slightly.

Perhaps you made it your mission to drop 30 pounds of body fat but are finding that after losing just 20, you're looking a little too thin. Now your goal changes and you want to build some muscle and fill out your frame.

This is why it's vital that you're always assessing your progress and re-evaluating the goals you have chosen for yourself. This will keep you right on track and striving for what's best moving into the future.

Rewards

Now, after you have your goals clearly set and outlined, next comes setting appropriate rewards. Rewards are going to be essential for enhancing the overall satisfaction that you get from obtaining those goals you set so they are not something to be looked over.

Rewards are typically based on two main principles – the principle to either gain pleasure or avoid pain. Usually when setting fitness rewards you'll be setting a reward that will allow you to gain pleasure so that's what you want to turn your focus to.

Rewards that are more centered around avoiding pain tend to be ones that are better used when you're trying to break bad habits (each time you eat a piece of chocolate you have to perform 50 push-ups).

When choosing your rewards to gain pleasure, always do try and avoid rewards that center around food however. Obviously you can go for the odd reward meal every now and then but if every reward you're after is based on food, you're not really enforcing the whole healthy lifestyle.

Whether it's a new CD to workout to or a new outfit to wear to the gym, select rewards that are important to you. Likely your short term rewards will be much smaller than your long term rewards, so keep that in mind also.

A long term reward could be a trip to some exotic location once you reach your goal weight and are confident to wear that bikini on the beach or go shirtless while relaxing by the pool.

Now let's move on and talk about what is necessary for fat loss to occur.

CHAPTER 6:
THE REQUIREMENTS FOR FAT LOSS

One big problem that many people face is that they never take the time to actually learn the requirements of proper fat loss. They'll go on some diet or workout plan that they've either been given by a trainer or that they've picked up in some magazine and just start going through it, hoping that it gives them the results that they are looking for.

While it's great that they are excited to be on their plan, it's very important that you're taking the time first to learn why fat loss happens.

When you can gain a better understanding of what causes the body to turn to body fat for fuel, you'll have a much better understanding of why you are or aren't seeing the results you should.

If you never truly realize what's going on while you're using this weight loss plan, there's a far greater chance that you'll find yourself lost.

Let's talk briefly about what fat loss is all about.

What Causes Weight Loss

Weight loss, by definition, is a very, very simple mathematical equation. Each and every day, your body is burning off calories. Some of these calories come from all the physical activity you do throughout the day and some of these calories come from physiological processes that go on in the body simply to keep you alive.

Generally speaking, your basal metabolic rate (BMR), which is how many calories your body would burn if you just sat in bed and didn't move a muscle (this is to keep your heart, lunges, brain, and other organs functioning properly), accounts for about 70% of the total calories you burn.

As you can see, this accounts for *a lot* of your daily expenditure. So right off the top, those that think you have to exercise to burn off fat are not quite correct. Your body will be burning off calories regardless of what you do just by being alive. Granted, minute for minute, you're obviously burning off *more* calories when you exercise than when you don't.

Second, the next component that accounts for how many calories you burn on a daily basis is the activity factor. This is basically how many calories you burn performing any physical task.

It could be cooking your breakfast in the morning, washing your hair in the shower, or going for a run after work. Anything that gets you moving goes into this category. As you can imagine, this is also the category that varies the most widely from individual to individual.

Someone who gets up and goes to work in an office all day, then resigns to the couch later that night for some good old reality TV is going to burn far fewer calories than someone who is going to a job where they are on their feet moving around all day long and then comes home and proceeds to hit the gym for a workout.

This second person would likely burn almost double the calories the sedentary person would over the course of the day so this will have a very large influence on their overall diet program set-up and how easily they are able to maintain their weight.

Finally, the last component that goes into determining how many calories you burn daily is what's called the 'thermic effect of food'. This essentially is how many calories your body burns off simply digesting the foods you eat.

For most people who are on a normal mixed diet, it will account for about 10% of their total calorie requirements. If you eat more protein in your diet however, you can actually increase this number and burn off more total calories over the course of the day.

If you eat 100 calories of pure protein for example, you're only going to 'net' (that is, total calories taken in minus total calories burned through digestion) about 70 calories.

Looking at carbohydrates and dietary fats on the other hand, if you take in 100 calories from those, you'll net 94 and 97 calories respectively.

While protein ramps the TEF up to 30%, carbs and fat only have a TEF of 6 and 3% respectively. So right there, simply by consuming a diet that contains more protein content, you can actually increase your daily calorie burn and speed up weight loss.

Obviously a 100% pure protein diet is never a good plan so don't take this too far, but focusing more of your food intake on these types of foods is a great idea when aiming for the goal of getting leaner.

With all of these factors added up – BMR, your activity burn, and TEF, you now have your *maintenance* calorie intake. This is how many calories you should eat each day if you want to stay exactly the same. You don't want to lose weight; you don't want to gain weight.

You're going to be in *balance*.

Now, if you aren't in balance, that's when you start to see some changes.

By looking at the picture below, you can see just how powerful altering this calorie balance can be. If you maintain the negative calorie balance, you're going to drop weight quickly like Sylvie below.

Or, if you're strength training and providing a slight calorie surplus, then you're going to see dramatic gains in muscle tissue like Angus. Remember how we talked about how muscle burns 35-50 calories per day? You can imagine just how much Angus who packed on 40 pounds of lean muscle is enjoying the benefits!

Angus:
I decided to try End Result Fitness because I was eating foods I hate and spending over 8 hours a week in the gym and not seeing any results. I was able to gain over 40 lbs of lean muscle and have seen more results in the past 4-6 months than I did in 5 years on my own. I'm now eating foods I love and only working out 3-4 times a week for 30 minutes each time. That's less than 2 hours a week!

Before | After | **GAINED 40 LBS OF LEAN MUSCLE**

Sylvie:
I decided to try End Result Fitness because I wanted to make healthy changes and I needed a plan that would fit in with my busy life. I was able to lose over 120 lbs of body fat and sculpt the slim, sexy body I've always wanted in just 12 short months. I'm now wearing clothes I love and my boyfriend can't stop complimenting my hot new body!

Before | After | **LOST 120 LBS OF BODY FAT**

Scott
I went from a weak and pudgy 185 lbs with 24% body fat to a lean and strong 165 lbs with only 12% body fat. I love that End Result Fitness completely transformed my body, health and quality of life.

Before | After | **LOST 12% BODY FAT**

The fact is, if you take in more calories through your food intake than your maintenance calorie intake, you've now provided the body with more energy than it needs. Since energy cannot be created or destroyed, the body has to do something with it. Thus, it converts it to body fat (or if you're doing a heavy resistance training program, some may be converted to muscle mass).

If, on the other hand, you take in fewer calories through your diet than you burn off over the course of the day, then you actually have to find energy from somewhere – namely, and hopefully, your body fat stores.

The problem is, it's not always just your body fat stores where this energy is found. And that is what we are about to discuss next.

What Causes Fat Loss

If you want to succeed at completely changing how you look, you don't just want to lose weight. No, you want to *lose fat*. There is a big difference between the two because one will just make you a smaller version of your current self and one will make you smaller, yet firmer.

If you're like most people, you're looking for the latter.

Losing body fat and losing body weight are very similar concepts in that you will still have to create that 'calorie deficit' (where you burn off more calories than you consume), the only thing is that you must be focusing on the types of foods you're eating as well as performing a proper exercise program in order to ensure that you keep your muscle mass and only burn off body fat.

Exercise plays an especially important role in this because if you're not exercising, your body sees no reason to hold onto your muscles, thus it's often the first tissue to get used up when searching for that added energy the body needs.

When you are exercising however, the body realizes that it must maintain this muscle to execute your daily tasks, therefore you are much more likely to utilize only body fat stores for fuel.

This is *much better*.

That is also why getting on a proper workout program by using End Result Fitness is going to mean the difference between losing weight and looking so-so and losing fat and looking like a brand new person.

When you work with us on a workout program designed especially for *fat loss* and for your specific body, you will change your body composition so you have more lean muscle mass and less fat mass. This is the win-win scenario you're after here. If you don't use a personalized program however, very rarely do you see these types of results occur.

How To Improve Fat Loss Naturally

Now, the final thing to note is that you can actually boost your ability to burn fat 24/7. Obviously in the ideal world this is what you want because then you're just burning off body fat all day long without doing a single thing. No extra exercise, no changes to your diet, you're just burning away calories at a higher rate than before.

Sound good?

No kidding. Now how do you go about doing this?

In order to turn your body into a calorie burning machine, what you want to focus on is increasing your BMR. Since, as we mentioned above, this accounts for up to 70% of the total daily calories that you burn off so by increasing this, you'll be really doing yourself a favour in the long run. Plus, since you will burn these calories off regardless of whether or not you're exercising, by increasing this you'll be really maximizing the fat loss that takes place each and every day.

There are a few methods of increasing your BMR.

1. First, you can maintain a regular exercise program. Simply by exercising you will increase your BMR over the long term. This is because as your body has to recover from all those exercise sessions, it's going to burn off more calories doing so.

So if you are making the effort to workout 3-5 days a week, you will naturally burn more calories all day long because of it. This is often referred to as the EPOC, which represents the fact that the body will be using more energy for an extended period of time once the workout has been completed.

2. The second and most effective way to boost your daily calorie burn is by adding more lean muscle mass to your body. This occurs as you complete a regular workout program that involves a strength component.

Think of it this way. Your fat mass burns about as much energy as a small Honda driving along the road. It gets great gas mileage and you can go a long way on little fuel.

For fat loss, this is precisely what you don't want. Good fuel mileage means it takes you hours to burn off hardly any calories and since total calories burned throughout the day is what will determine how quickly fat loss takes place, you can see how this works directly against you.

Your muscle mass however, unlike your fat mass, is about as fuel efficient as a mustang. Not only does it require higher quality fuel but it also burns it off twice as fast.

THIS is what you want your body to be like. Fuel inefficient. You want to be burning calories like crazy even while you're just sitting on the couch relaxing after a hard day at work.

Adding more muscle mass to your frame will do just that.

Let's give you some numbers here to really drive this notion home.

For every pound of lean muscle mass you build, that pound will require an additional 50-75 *calories per day* just to stay there. This is how much fuel it burns just maintaining the tissues, not doing any work.

Each pound of fat you have burns about 2 calories per day. See the difference?

Obviously, having more muscle mass as opposed to more fat mass is going to work hugely in your favour. If you can add just ten pounds of muscle to your body, that could mean burning off an additional 500 calories or more each and every day. *Without any additional work.*

Think about it this way. If you burned off 500 calories more per day without doing anything else different right now, that would equal 3500 calories per week. How many calories are in one pound of body fat? *3500!* Simply by adding that lean muscle tissue you will lose one pound of body fat each week. This is basically getting your body to do the fat loss work for you.

If that doesn't get you to sit up and get you interested, I'm not sure what will. By far this is *the* most effective approach to seeing the body that you want.

As you can see, those two methods actually work with each other as well – you have to exercise to build the muscle tissue, you'll naturally get a higher metabolic rate because of that fact and then once that tissue is built, you'll maintain that higher metabolic rate over the long term.

This is the primary factor that we really focus on at End Result Fitness. Since we know you obviously don't want to reach your goal weight only to have that weight come back on in a short period of time, we're driven to ensuring that it stays off for good.

By setting you up with a skyrocket metabolic rate, you will have no problem maintaining your body weight and your body fat loss once you've stopped the fat loss diet and are moving into a stage of maintenance.

Even if you do happen to cheat on your diet every now and then, it won't affect you like how it used to because you'll be burning up calories so quickly each and every day.

This is really the difference between success and failure for most people. The rebound rate after fat loss is incredibly, INCREDIBLY high and this is why.

These dieters don't take the time to focus on increasing their BMR, so as soon as they go off that program and start reverting to their old ways, that weight comes right back on.

Since when you use an intensely restricted calorie intake your metabolic rate is naturally going to slow, when you come off it then you're going to notice that it's far easier to start gaining body fat.

If you come off your diet with a metabolism so slow it's hardly running at all, how do you expect to maintain the weight loss?

You won't.

Here is a graphical image that explains this concept nicely.

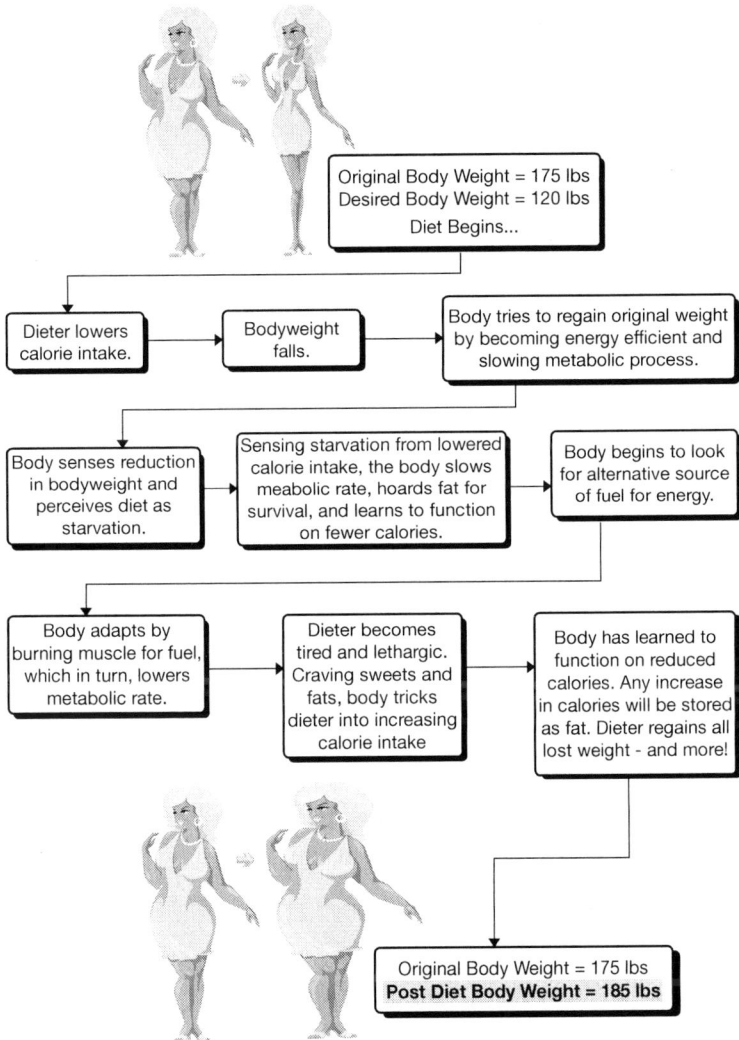

Your Body's Defense Mechanism Against Dieting or Starvation

Original Body Weight = 175 lbs
Desired Body Weight = 120 lbs
Diet Begins...

Dieter lowers calorie intake. → Bodyweight falls. → Body tries to regain original weight by becoming energy efficient and slowing metabolic process.

Body senses reduction in bodyweight and perceives diet as starvation. → Sensing starvation from lowered calorie intake, the body slows meabolic rate, hoards fat for survival, and learns to function on fewer calories. → Body begins to look for alternative source of fuel for energy.

Body adapts by burning muscle for fuel, which in turn, lowers metabolic rate. → Dieter becomes tired and lethargic. Craving sweets and fats, body tricks dieter into increasing calorie intake → Body has learned to function on reduced calories. Any increase in calories will be stored as fat. Dieter regains all lost weight - and more!

Original Body Weight = 175 lbs
Post Diet Body Weight = 185 lbs

This is the unavoidable result of "restricted calorie" diets!

STOP Yo-Yo Dieting

Obviously, we are going to set you up on a realistic lifestyle plan so you don't revert to your old ways. You will find this plan more than doable since you'll be taking in plenty of delicious food and burning more of it off each and every day.

Now let's start getting into the details you've really been waiting for, the nutritional principles you need to know to see maximum fat loss.

SECTION 2:
NUTRITIONAL PRINCIPLES FOR OPTIMAL FAT LOSS

Earlier we have discussed the main concepts that need to be at play in order for fat loss to take place. The one element that can very easily make or break your program is the diet that you're following. If you don't have a proper fat loss diet laid out, you're going to be hard pressed to see the results you're after.

Unfortunately, there are so many different fat loss diets out there that it can be incredibly hard to weed through them all and find out which ones work and which don't.

Luckily, I'm about to share with you all the essential information that you need to know so that you never have to follow one of those diets again. Instead, you'll be focused on proper eating strategies that will help the fat just melt off all without having to count every single calorie that you consume.

While it is important that you are monitoring how much food you're eating and have some degree of calorie awareness as this will play a role in how you progress with your weight loss, you don't have to go off and become a human calculator either. Doing so would just cause unnecessary stress to your day and make it that much more likely that you fall off your program altogether.

So let's dive in and begin discussing the most important information you must know about eating for optimal fat loss.

CHAPTER 7:
WHY NUTRITION IS SO IMPORTANT FOR FAT LOSS

In the introduction we covered just how important nutrition is when it comes to fat loss. By why is it so important? Couldn't you just get away with exercising more and not change the way you eat?

The reason nutrition is so important when you're looking to achieve maximum fat loss is because first, as we eluded to when speaking of how fat loss occurs, your nutritional intake will in part determine whether or not you lose weight or you lose fat.

If you want to look your best, fat loss is what you're after. Nutrition, which is going to be making sure you get the right combination of nutrients to the body will go a long way towards ensuring that you're getting that proper mix of nutrients that protects those muscle tissues.

Secondly, the next reason why nutrition is so vital is because it's far easier to create that calorie deficit through food than it is through exercise.

Put it this way, the average person who goes out and runs for one hour will burn approximately 500-700 calories depending on how intensely they are running.

Now, if you were to eat just one slice of cheesecake, you'd take in approximately 500-800 calories, depending on the type and the size. How long does it take you to eat that cheesecake?

3 minutes? 5 minutes? 1 minute if it's your absolute favorite variety?

It is so easy to overconsume in calories yet so hard to burn those calories off. If you were to eat to your heart's content and just try and burn off all those calories, you might as well chain yourself to a treadmill all night long because all your free time would be spent there.

Far too many people underestimate just how much time is needed exercising in order to burn off the foods they consume so they end up running into major problems as far as fat loss goes. They think that they're burning up hundreds upon hundreds of calories with each workout session they do when they're really doing anything but that.

If you can control your diet intake, then you're going to see far quicker progress reaching your fat loss goals.

The Problem With Most Diets

When it comes to most diet plans, there are a few major problems that you'll run into. By being able to identify what these problems are, you're much better able to pinpoint exactly what you must do to overcome them and get yourself right back on track again.

Let's have a look at the major issues that tend to occur.

Too Low Of Calories

The very first issue that you'll cross with some diets is that they are far too low in overall calorie content. Ever come across a plan that provided fewer than 1000 calories?

If so, that should have been immediately crossed off your list. You have to remember that while lower calories is good, extremely low calories is not good.

The lower your calorie intake the greater the chances that you're going to experience a slowed metabolic rate and further issues maintaining fat loss in the long run. Your body senses that you're trying to starve it and because of this, it slows everything way down.

As it does this, it's also going to start burning off lean muscle tissue which, as we've touched upon earlier, is the tissue that is like your calorie-burning engine. The more of it you have, the faster you burn off body fat. As soon as you start losing lean muscle tissue, you're going to struggle to keep losing weight.

The body realizes that muscle tissue is the most 'costly' tissue to maintain and because of that, it has a better chance of survival without it. Hence you lose lean body mass.

Therefore, it's a fine line that you have to be on. You don't want to consume too few calories because that sends the wrong signal to the body but you can't consume too many otherwise you won't cause fat loss to happen.

Any diet that has you eating fewer than 1000 calories however is neither sound nor smart. All it will do is mess up your health and metabolism in the future.

Lack Of Variety

Second, the next problem with many diets today is that they offer very little variety.

Breakfast is a bowl of bran cereal, a piece of fruit, and eggs.

Lunch is a salad with some chicken and maybe a banana if you're lucky.

Your snack consists of a handful of almonds with some yogurt.

Dinner is white fish with steamed vegetables.

And your before bed snack, if you're lucky enough to have one, is nothing more than a few saltine crackers or a half a cup of grapes.

It's nothing but bland and boring. Day in and day out.

If you want to stick with your diet in the long haul, you need to ensure there is enough variety to keep you satisfied. As long as you're choosing healthy foods and meeting your nutrient and calorie requirements, there's no reason to confine yourself to the same old four or five meals week after week after week.

Diets that do offer more variety and choice tend to be far better for most people since we as humans naturally crave variety. You can't get past the fact that we do partly eat for pleasure sake and if you aren't giving your body this pleasure from food in your meals, eventually you will cheat.

Plain and simple.

No Type Of Metabolic Prevention Strategy

Third, another huge issue that most popular mainstream diets face is that they give very little information in the way of a metabolic preventative strategy. What this essentially means is that despite the fact that you are using a lower calorie intake, the diet you're on has no way of protecting against or preventing the reduced metabolic rate that naturally comes with this type of diet.

So while you may see results on it for the first few weeks while your body is adapting, once that initial time period has passed, those results fail to continue. Your body has now adapted to this reduced calorie intake and has slowed down how many calories it burns on a daily basis because of it (that BMR value we discussed earlier).

So now you're stuck with two options.

1. Abandon the diet altogether – which, obviously if you're set on losing weight is not an option.

2. Reduce your calories further yet, hoping that starts getting fat loss moving.

You may decide to opt for choice two, reducing your calories by another couple hundred a day, but in two more weeks, you're back facing the same situation. You did move ahead and lost another pound or two after that cut back, but now you've hit plateau just like before only now you are consuming *fewer* calories than you were before.

G-R-E-A-T.

So again, you have two options.

1. Abandon the diet altogether – which, now may be starting to seem like a mighty fine option (your stomach is hardly satisfied on the half a plate of food you're consuming).

2. Decrease those calories again.

The brave souls – the ones who are determined to have success – will likely choose option two. So off they go, reducing back their calories. Again, they see another pound or two lost but then get stuck again.

This is an endless cycle that is absolutely disastrous to get into because it means that you'll eventually wind up eating so few calories and losing very little weight because of it.

Obviously since you can't subside on no food you can only take this so far before you have to come off it – you have no other option.

But, what a proper diet plan will have is safeguards to protect against this. On an effective diet plan your metabolism will never slow down like it did in the above scenario, so you won't have to worry about hitting that dreaded plateau and when you do, the plan provides immediately strategies for how to get out of it.

That is what defines a good diet.

So there you have some of the main problems that occur with most diet plans. Fortunately, with the diet plan we've created we've overcome all of these hurdles so you don't have to suffer any of their ill effects.

Now let's move on and start discussing some of the biggest diet myths that are out there.

If you're planning on attempting fat loss, you must pay attention to these ones.

CHAPTER 8:
THE BIGGEST DIET MYTHS

Over the years, there are numerous diet myths that have all come to be either passed around by mouth to mouth from one dieter to the other or broadcasted to the mainstream media by celebrities or popular 'health' authorities.

Unfortunately, many of these myths are just going to lead you incredibly astray and do nothing but harm your progress in the long run. Let's go over a few of the more major ones that you must know so you can get a better sense for what *not* to do while on your diet plan.

Eating Before Bed Automatically Makes You Gain Weight

The very first myth that often circulates and one that far too many people believe is that if they eat something late at night, it doesn't matter what it is, it's going straight to their hips.

While there is some truth to that statement, it's far from being entirely correct.

The problem that occurs with late night eating is not the fact that you're eating, it's more what you are eating and what that food causes you to do.

Think about it for a second. When you reach into the pantry at 10:30 pm looking for a snack, what are you likely to come up with?

It's not lean protein or vegetables. It's more along the lines of chips, chocolate, cookies, snack crackers, popcorn, and so on. The foods you eat late at night are naturally sugar and calorie filled as this is what we've been taught 'snack' foods are. It doesn't help the situation that we are exposed to commercial after commercial while watching TV to prompt us to go reaching for a snack just like this.

But yet that's what we grab and these snacks do one thing. *Encourage you to eat more.*

Because of the actual make-up of these snack foods (high in processed, simple carbs) they will send insulin levels skyrocketing and then dropping faster than a penny tossed off the top of the Eiffel Tower. As this drop occurs you're left with rebound hunger that sends you running right back into that pantry in search of more.

This cycle continues on and on until you go to bed and before you know it, you've consumed upwards of 600 calories.

Now unless those 600 calories were already factored into your fat loss diet menu, you're going to likely gain weight because of it.

Remember that calorie balance equation for fat loss – more calories burned off than consumed through food? Well, with that 600 calorie 'snack' you just ate as the clock approaches midnight, you've cancelled out whatever deficit you did have going on and now have eaten your way into what could very well be, *weight gain.*

So this is the real reason why late-night eating tends to make us gain weight. It's not because we are eating – if you choose a healthy snack and make sure to plan for those calories so they are a natural part of your daily intake then there should be no problem including them into your day without seeing weight gain.

The key is food selection and moderation when it comes to serving size. If you can get both of these right then you're on your way to success.

Eating Foods In Certain Combinations Will Be Better For Fat Loss

Another common fat loss myth that you'll often hear circulating around is that if you eat certain foods in combination with each other, that will help you lose weight faster.

Often these are referred to as 'food combining diets'. They state that if you eat A with B and never X then you should see Y weight loss. Confused?

You should be. Usually these types of diets are not based on any form of actual science and are quite simply just going to lead you astray.

The one exception to this rule is diets that state you should always eat protein with your carbohydrates and fats. This is a fact and is true. Protein should be included in each and every snack or meal you eat since it really is like the cornerstone of your diet.

But diets that give specific reference as to actual food pairings (grapefruits can go with wheat toast but never eat an orange with that toast or it's trouble) are nothing more than voodoo magic. Don't fall for them because all they may provide you with is a bit of a mental workout trying to figure out what the heck you actually can eat.

There Are 'Negative Calorie Foods'

Another common myth that you may find yourself believing is that there's such a thing as negative calorie foods. What this myth states is that by eating a particular food, you're actually going to be burning off more calories in doing so than what you're consuming. So the theory is that by eating these foods you'll actually lose weight.

Eat to lose weight? Sounds a little too good to be true.

And it is.

There is no such thing as a negative calorie food. Yes, celery comes close but the fact of the matter is that you will never burn off more calories digesting a food than you did while you consumed it. There is just no way of this ever being possible.

It is true that there are plenty of foods out there that contain so few calories when you factor in fiber and the total water content that there's really no reason to even add these to your daily calorie intake (such as celery, cabbage, lettuce, broccoli, etc). None of these foods will make you lose weight just by eating them.

Waiting To Eat Breakfast Boosts Your Chances Of Success

How many times have you heard someone say they're skipping breakfast because they're watching their weight?

Too many times to count? Chances are you have heard this exact phrase before many, many times.

Often people will think that if they want to lose weight quicker, that's the thing to do. Skip the first meal so they're already burning off their body fat stores and helping bring their total calorie intake down a notch.

The problem here is that this more often than not fails horribly. What happens is that while you may feel fine for the first hour or so in the morning, eventually it hits you.

You haven't had any food to eat and are asking your body to function optimally and it becomes *starved*. And, if you've ever experienced extreme hunger like you're going to see in this scenario, that type of hunger is next to impossible to control. So there you go, off to look for the fastest source of fuel that you can find – which, just happens to come from the vending machine or local coffee house more often than not.

So rather than eating a nice 200-300 calorie breakfast that was well balanced and supplied your body with nutrients, you'll polish off a few donuts, a bagel with cream cheese, or a chocolate bar and a bag of Skittles, all setting you back 400 calories or more.

Now how are you doing in your progress towards weight loss? Starving yourself right at the start of the day is never a wise move and it will almost always come back to get you as time goes on. Instead, fuel your body right.

When you give it a good breakfast you stroke the metabolic engine and increase the chances that you see fat loss taking place.

Remember, when you wake up in the morning your body has been fasting over the entire course of the night. For most of you this adds up to six to eight hours without any food whatsoever and the body is crying out for nutrition.

If you don't consume breakfast, you'll just be setting yourself up to see a reduced metabolic rate over the coming day making fat loss progress more difficult.

Get up and eat breakfast – it's the best way to jumpstart your metabolism and set you up for good calorie burning all day long.

Waiting To Eat After Exercise Increases Fat Burning

Along with skipping your breakfast meal, another common misconception that some people have about the process of dieting is that if they wait to eat after a workout is completed they will increase the chances that they burn off additional body fat from that workout itself.

The thought process is that now that they have the body in 'fat burning mode' if they begin to eat again they take it right out of it and hence, stop their progress.

What you must realize here is that while you may get your body burning off fat as fuel, it's still that total number at the end of the day that matters. If you consume more calories than you burned off over the course of the day, it doesn't matter how much 'fat' you burned off, you'll still gain weight.

This is why some people who workout very hard and then treat themselves later on in the day since they did put in such a good workout don't see success.

Even though they may have burned off fat during the workout, since they consumed junk food later on in the day, they ended up putting that fat right back on.

Remember you must fuel your muscles properly for exercise but then also keep fuelling them properly throughout the day.

It all comes down to that balance, so don't let yourself think that by eating immediately after a workout you are shorting your results. If the truth is told by doing so you're actually increasing your results since then you will be making sure that the muscles are recovered well so you can work harder again next workout.

This hard work will then increase your basal metabolic rate even further, causing that much more fat loss. It's a really great cycle to be in – these increases to your basal metabolic rate and as soon as you get on with the process of building more muscle tissue, you're going to reap all the rewards of it and move you closer to your *end result*.

Your muscles are especially ready to take up nutrients that you feed them immediately after a workout session and if you miss this opportunity, you won't recover as fast and you may not get the results you should be from that workout session.

Immediately after exercise is one of the most important times of the day to be eating so be sure that you don't skip it.

To Lose Fat Avoid Eating Fat

While it's not as common any more, there are still plenty of people out there who have some type of 'fat phobia'. To them, they believe that if they eat dietary fat, this is going to cause them to gain body fat. After all, if you eat fat, you gain fat, right?

Again, this is incorrect. Dietary fat does not directly go straight to body fat when you eat it. It's true that there is a higher chance it will go to body fat if you are consuming too many calories simply because the body has no storage capacity with this nutrient like it does for carbohydrates (which get stored as something called 'muscle glycogen'), but even still, if you're making sure your calorie level is where it needs to be, it's perfectly possible to consume dietary fat without it turning to fat.

Then it will be used for the vital functions that the body needs it for in order to survive and it will also be used up for energy. In fact, many people who consume some dietary fat in their diet show greater results than those who are consuming virtually no fat at all.

Dietary fat is a very healthy part of a well-rounded diet and some should be present in your plan at all times.

It's the type and the amount that matters – two issues that we'll be discussing more closely later on.

Carbs Are Evil – Avoid At All Costs

Second, another common notion that some people will come to believe is that carbohydrates, any way you slice them, are evil. To them, carbs are a group of food that will make you fat – no matter what.

It doesn't take much to realize that low-carb diets are all the rage right now. All you have to do is walk into a supermarket and scan the popular magazines to see low carb headlines gracing the covers.

Everywhere you turn people seem to be adopting this diet strategy thinking it's the one that will finally help them shed their weight. And for some people, it very well may be.

There are many benefits to using a lower carb diet approach such as reduced hunger levels and a better ability to control calorie intake but that said, there's nothing 'magical' about low carb dieting.

Some people mistakenly believe that when they eat low carb they put their body into some type of special circumstance where it's burning up faster than ever before.

This is very incorrect. If the truth was told, low carb dieting actually *increases* your risk for that metabolism slow-down phenomenon that we discussed earlier (remember, the one where the dieter either had to continually lower her calorie intake or abandon the diet completely). In theory you stand more of a chance of having problems on this diet than on any other diet out there.

When done correctly though you can obviously prevent this from taking place and ensure that the diet does work for you. The point is that you just shouldn't place carbohydrates on the 'ban' list for no reason.

These can very easily – and very well should – be added to a healthy weight loss diet plan.

As Long As You Eat Healthy, You Can Eat However Much You Want

Moving on, our last dietary myth that you should be keeping in mind is the myth that 'as long as it's healthy, you can eat however much of it you want'.

The person who believes this myth is the person who goes off eating like crazy on all the healthy food they can get their hands on. They eat bowls and bowls of whole grain cereal, loads of fruits for their snacks, and a whole tub of low-fat yogurt for a bed-time snack because they believe all of these foods are healthy for them.

And very likely they are. But the point this person misses is the fact that even though they are healthy, they still contribute calories to their day.

Remember that calorie balance equation? We do keep referring back to this but that's simply because it is THAT important; all other factors pale in comparison when referring to maximum fat loss. If you can't get that calorie balance under control, you aren't going to be seeing fat loss take place.

Even if you're eating nothing but carrots and fish – if you eat too much of it, you'll gain weight.

Your chances of consuming far too many calories from healthy foods are a lot lower than they are if you were eating unhealthy foods since most unhealthy foods are much more calorie dense (have more calories per volume of food), but still, if you're a determined eater with a big appetite, it is extremely possible to eat too many calories of healthy foods.

Just ask any one of the 'healthy eaters' you see on the street who is still overweight.

So there you have the main diet myths that you must make yourself aware of. By equipping yourself with this information you ensure that you stay on top of the fat loss game and that you're making the most out of your diet to see results.

Failing to keep track of these myths and falling for even just one will have an influence on the overall results you see.

Now let's move forward and start working out the specifics of your diet plan.

CHAPTER 9:
ALL ABOUT PROTEIN

Now, before we dive in and give you some thorough information on the various types of macronutrients, I want to stress right now that the whole point of this is not to turn you into some meticulous calorie counting machine.

You can certainly do that if you wish but the vast majority of people will find that tedious, frustrating, and just leaving them wishing they could abandon their diet altogether.

Instead, we're going to educate you on roughly how many calories you should be shooting for each day so you can get a general idea of what this looks like in food on a day to day basis.

This way, you can do a bit of research up on some of the foods you enjoy eating on your plan so you can see the general recommended amounts of them and how they will go about fitting into your diet.

This should give you a very good basis of understanding that you can then use to help you navigate throughout your plan.

Obviously since your activity levels will vary somewhat on a day to day basis it's impossible to ever be 100% certain of what your calorie needs are but if you give yourself a range of say 100-150 calories either way, you should be hitting it fairly close to spot on.

If you think back to when you took your initial stats, you will have already figured out your *target fat loss calorie intake*, so now that you already have this all lined up, you're going to be assessing how much of each type of food to be eating.

This is important for ensuring fat loss takes place and also making certain that you get all the nutrients you require for overall good nutrition. If you fail to eat the right combinations of foods throughout the diet, you may find that you aren't progressing as well as you should.

So all of this said, now let's dive in and begin talking a little bit about protein.

Protein is by far the single most important nutrient for you to be taking in on your diet on a regular basis. It's essentially a part of the integral structure of every single tissue on your body and fuels all the major processes that go on to sustain life. Without enough protein, you would eventually become malnourished and die. THAT is how important it is.

Unfortunately, many people aren't even coming close to meeting their needs, which is a big reason why they aren't losing weight like they should.

For the average person, approximately one gram of protein per pound of bodyweight is what is required if you're leading an active lifestyle. If you aren't exercising you may be able to get away with slightly less than this just since you won't have the demands on the muscle tissues like that of which you do when you are being so active.

When you're aiming for fat loss however, you'll want to boost this intake up even higher. The reason for this is because as you drop your calorie intake, you're essentially giving the body less energy to use for fuel.

Since it's going to always use incoming fuel first for energy rather than diving straight for your body fat stores, there is a very good chance that some of the protein that you eat from food will actually get broken down and used for energy, rather than being used for its primary purposes (repairing and maintaining lean muscle, as well as all the other tissues in the body). So if you were only taking in just your one gram/lb figure, you may use a quarter to a half of this strictly for energy purposes.

Now where does that leave you in terms of available protein for maintaining your lean muscle?

It leaves you short. You simply will not have enough protein necessary to see proper results. This is why when dieting, we increase your protein up even higher – this way, if you do use some for fuel, you have plenty left over to spare for your lean muscle mass.

Remember, our primary focus during a fat loss phase is to keep that lean muscle you have. This is the tissue that strokes your BMR and will make it that much easier to continue to lose fat and keep it off over the long run. Everything we do is based on that concept so it's why you're going to hear me talking about it so much.

The better protein intake when dieting will be closer to 1.25 to 1.5 grams of protein per pound. This may seem like a lot to you but if you're eating the proper foods, then it'll add up very quickly.

What foods are your best sources of protein?

Ideally you want to look for lean sources of pure protein such as:

- Chicken breasts
- White turkey meat
- Ground lean turkey breast
- Eggs and egg whites
- Fish
- Seafood (shrimp, crab, lobster)
- Lean cuts of red meat
- Vension
- Whey protein powder
- Skim milk
- Low-fat cheese, which needs to be 4% milk fat or less
- Greek yogurt
- Low-fat cottage cheese
- Tofu
- High quality soy protein
- High quality whey protein

These are all going to supply you with the essential amino acids your muscles need and deliver a whole host of other good nutrients.

The protein choices that you want to stay away from as they either contain too much saturated fat or have far too many additives to be healthy include:

- Bacon
- Sausage
- Sandwich meat (very high in sodium)
- Ground beef
- Salami
- Beef jerky (very high in sodium so eat on occasion only)
- High fat milk and or dairy products

While these do contain some protein, they just are not your best options so it's best to stay clear whenever possible.

In addition to supporting all the main body functions that we outlined earlier, protein also offers a number of advantages. Let's take a look.

1. Increased Satiety

One of the biggest benefits for upping your protein intake while on a fat loss diet plan is because out of all the three macronutrients, protein tends to leave you feeling the fullest immediately after consuming it.

So if you fill your plate with a larger serving of protein and a smaller serving of carbohydrates, you're going to find that you keep your hunger levels much more constant after the meal is finished and are far less likely to go in for seconds.

One good tip is to try eating your protein at the start of the meal if you can so you get these satiety benefits right away. By beginning with it you may just find that you're a lot less tempted to continue on eating after having finished that thus you'll naturally take in fewer calories at that particular meal.

2. Increased Thermic Effect Of Food

Second, another huge benefit of protein when it comes to fat loss is that eating it supercharges your metabolism.

Remember that thermic effect of food factor we discussed earlier? This was how many calories your body burned off simply digesting the foods you eat.

Well, protein rates the highest. If you recall for every 100 calories of pure protein you take in, you'll burn off about 30 of those calories just digesting it.

It's like getting a mini-workout in itself! So if you want an instant boost to your metabolic rate, focus on protein. It will accomplish this for you.

3. Slows Digestion

Third, the final thing that protein will help you out with is that it will slow down the digestion process. While it burns off the most calories through digestion, it also takes the longest as the body has to work hard to break all the amino acids down and send them off to their various places in the body to execute tasks.

Normally, when you take in carbohydrates at a meal, your insulin levels will quickly increase and the body will take these carbs immediately out of the blood stream and either use them for fuel or deposit them in storage.

But, when protein is present, this process doesn't happen so quickly so for that reason, those carbohydrates won't get tucked into body fat stores as readily, thus you'll have a lower chance of gaining body fat at that particular meal.

Always pairing your carbohydrates with your protein is one of the best things that you can do to ensure that you feel great after every meal you consume.

So there you have some of the main benefits of protein. As you can see this type of food has a lot to offer the fat loss enthusiast and is definitely an important part of your day.

Before we leave off on protein we should just make mention of those who wish to lead a vegetarian lifestyle. This is becoming more and more popular in today's times and it's definitely doable to lose weight just as well being a vegetarian than not.

What you will have to make sure of if you plan to maintain a vegetarian diet is that you are taking the time to carefully plan out your protein intake. For you, some pre-planning will definitely be required in the diet because without it, the chances that you do short yourself on your intake will be very high.

Many of the foods vegetarians tend to lean towards are lower on the protein end of the scale so without some type of regulation, you could be in for a few problems.

Some good sources of protein to include in the vegetarian diet are:

- Beans and legumes
- Nuts and seeds
- Tempeh
- Soy
- Tofu
- Seaweed
- Higher protein vegetables

In some instances certain vegetarians may also consume dairy products or seafood/fish just depending on the exact specific type of vegetarian they are.

If you do consume dairy and eggs, that will definitely open up more options for you in terms of getting your protein intake since low-fat dairy is so high in protein as are egg whites.

Likewise, if you'll eat fish on your diet, again, you'll have no trouble meeting your protein intake since fish is such a high-quality, concentrated form of protein.

If you don't though and you are a strict vegetarian, just plan your meals properly and you should still be able to reach that one gram per pound intake, if not slightly higher to make it even better for fat loss purposes.

Now let's move on and talk a little more about carbohydrates.

CHAPTER 10:
ALL ABOUT CARBOHYDRATES

Without question, carbohydrates are the nutrient that is most often debated and questioned within the context of fat loss and even weight maintenance for that matter.

Many people are currently very confused on what the verdict is on protein. Is it helpful for weight loss or harmful?

If you feel like your head is spinning at the thought of even thinking about what carbohydrates to eat and how much in order to see fat loss progress, you aren't alone. Most people feel this exact same way which is why it's so vital to set the record straight once and for all.

Carbohydrates themselves, do not make you gain body fat any faster than protein or dietary fat would, apart from possibly the TEF factor. Just like protein, carbohydrates contain four calories per gram (remember fat contains nine) so gram for gram they don't actually put more body fat on you.

The problem that some people experience with carbohydrates though and what causes them to make you gain body fat is the fact that they will increase hunger levels after eating them, therefore making you want to eat more food.

If you aren't keeping a close eye on your calorie intake, it's then very easy to go over your target fat loss calorie intake that we discussed earlier and that's when you'll see issues with progress.

Not all carbohydrates will spark high levels of hunger (which we'll go over in a minute) but many do and you must be aware of that.

Plus, many people also misjudge how much carbs their eating so that also factors into the equation. They'll sit down to a bowl of pasta and think they're only eating a couple servings of carbs when really it's more like 5-8 servings in that meal alone. Because this perception of portion size is so skewed, it's very easy to completely eliminate a daily deficit right there in that single meal.

That's not to mention cereals, breads, crackers, granola bars, and all the other carb-rich foods that are easy to underestimate as well.

Fructose Versus Glucose

Something else that you must keep in mind when it comes to carbohydrates is the different between fructose and glucose. These are both forms of carbohydrates however their individual chemical make-up is slightly different meaning they will have differing impacts on the body's tissues.

If you don't understand the difference, it could potentially have a very devastating impact on your diet progress.

What you need to know is that upon consumption, fructose is immediately transferred over to the liver tissues rather than going into the blood stream like glucose is.

High glucose foods (such as candy, cakes, cookies, etc) will move right into your blood, producing that blood sugar spike followed by the crash that we discussed earlier. If you do happen to need energy at that point however, or if the storage form of carbohydrates in the muscle cells (called muscle glycogen) does happen to be depleted, then rather than converting these carbohydrates straight to body fat, they will be used for those purposes.

Since the more lean muscle mass you have, the more storage of carbohydrates will be necessary. This actually can make a significant influence over how easily you gain body fat. If you have plenty of muscle, you can afford to eat more glucose-based carbohydrates without seeing that resulting fat gain (yet ANOTHER reason to focus on building muscle!).

Glucose based carbohydrates also include foods such as bread, cereals (most), pasta, and rice. All of these hit the bloodstream and go from there.

Fructose on the other hand, as we mentioned, is sent off to the liver. The liver unfortunately has a very limited storage capacity for carbohydrates and is set at about 50 grams per day. So as soon as you pass this 50 gram threshold, any carbohydrates will be converted directly into body fat.

This is a big reason why there is so much noise being made about products that contain high fructose corn syrup (or HFCS). These foods are readily converted right into body fat, often as fast or faster than eating foods high in saturated fat.

Foods that typically contain fructose to be on the lookout for are:

- Soda
- Ketchup
- Some forms of candy
- Honey
- Maple syrup
- Processed snack foods
- Fruits

Now, fruits are on this list because they are in fact half fructose and half glucose. But does that mean you should go off avoiding fruit altogether?

Not quite. The important thing to know here is that fruits only contain about 5-10 grams of fructose each so they really aren't going to do a lot of harm *unless* you are consuming upwards of 10 pieces of fruit per day or are eating a diet that is high in fructose from other foods.

Then you may see resulting fat gain but one or two fruits added to your day if you are sure to stay away with anything that contains HFCS will not be a problem.

What's better is the fact that fruits contain many essential nutrients that you do need on a daily basis and will also not boost your blood sugar levels like some other more refined-carbohydrate glucose based snacks will.

For that reason people tend to find that eating fruit fills them up quickly and keeps them satisfied. They have plenty of fiber as well, which is an essential nutrient to slow down the digestion of food and passage through your system.

So there you have the big difference between glucose and fructose. This is vital to know because it will impact how you progress on your diet.

It would be a very wise move to start scanning every ingredient listing on the products you buy to look for the words 'fructose' high-fructose corn syrup', or even, 'high glucose-fructose corn syrup'. If you see these words anywhere listed, put that product back on the self. It's not for you.

Note too that often this isn't listed on the actual nutrition chart given so you'll have to go through reading the ingredient listing itself to search for whether it contains fructose.

Most often carbohydrates are either listed as a whole or will be subdivided between sugar and dietary fiber.

Fructose and glucose are not separated out so you'll have to use a bit of detective work here to figure out if the product in fact contains it.

Now let's talk a little more about that 'low carb diet' that everyone seems to be jumping on.

Low-Carb Diets

Do you shutter at the mere mention of low carb dieting? Many people do because let's face it, carbs are tasty. Carbohydrates actually cause the body to release serotonin which is the 'feel good hormone' that is actually also released when using some recreational (and illegal) drugs. So it makes sense that we as humans naturally tend to want carbs – they make us feel good.

In addition to that, carbs are the preferred source of fuel for the body so any time your body is lacking fuel (such as when on a diet) carbs are what it craves.

Now if you're someone who really, really dislikes the thought of cutting carbs out of their meal plan, chances are low carb dieting isn't for you. You'll have craving after craving after craving and just end up falling off the plan.

If you feel as though you could 'take it or leave it' when it comes to carbs, then low carb dieting may be something for you to look into.

Just note that you don't need to reduce carbs entirely to lose weight. Far too many people believe it's the only way to go and this is not the case at all.

In fact, I would never recommend cutting carbohydrates out entirely as they do supply vital nutrients that you do require for life (especially vegetables) and you require some carbohydrates each day if you hope to maintain any intensity with your workouts – and I hope you do.

But, I do believe that *moderating* your carbohydrate is a good thing. You'll find you get less hungry on the diet (due to steadier levels of blood sugar and less of an insulin release) and you'll also do away with any bloating that often comes from carbohydrates. Some people really do notice that they puff up after eating certain carb based foods so on a low carb diet, you can deal with this quite nicely.

One of the primary reasons also that I suggest never lowering your carbohydrates too far is because there are a few big problems with low carb diets in general.

Let's have a quick look at what a few of these are.

1. Slowed Metabolism

The very first problem that you may encounter while on a low carb fat loss diet is that you'll have an increased risk of suffering from a slow metabolism.

This is due to the fact that since carbohydrates are the primary macronutrient that will stroke the metabolic rate, when you're low in them for extended periods of time, this has implications on how fast your body burns off energy.

This is all related to a certain hormone in the body referred to as 'Leptin', which essentially monitors both the incoming food intake as well as what your current body fat levels are.

If you start to decrease your food intake dramatically or you begin to approach extremely low body fat levels (lower than what the body would ideally like you to be at), that's when you're going to find that you see these Leptin levels changing from their normal concentrations in the body and that your weight loss progress comes screeching to a halt.

Leptin is a very intensely regulated hormone in the body and when concentration levels do alter, you're going to notice signs and symptoms such as intense hunger, very low energy levels, a feeling of being cold all the time, and a strong urge to eat.

This is the body's natural way of preventing starvation from taking place as it's doing everything it can to prompt you to eat. At this point, you have to fight extremely hard to stick with your diet and most people will find that they do actually just fall off the plan altogether.

In order to overcome this problem, high carbohydrate feedings have to be introduced into the low carbohydrate diet which counteracts the effects of these altered Leptin levels and returns them closer to normal again.

2. Low Energy Levels

Second, another big problem with the low carb diets is that they will provoke very low energy levels. If you've ever cut out all your carbs suddenly from your diet, you can see very well how predominant this is.

For the first day or two you may be fine as your body still has enough built-up storage of carbohydrates to keep you going but after that, you're going to be suffering. Fatigue hits in and getting to the gym seems harder and harder and pretty soon, your activity levels drop dramatically.

This can obviously have a big influence over how many calories you're burning on a daily basis and is another thing that will offset fat loss from occurring.

Fortunately, if you do stick with the low carb diet long enough you'll often see this problem clearing up somewhat as the body adapts to this type of diet, but if you want to keep up your workouts, you will still have to be adding carbohydrates at one point or another. If you don't, you simply cannot expect to continue with your weight lifting sessions.

3. Adherence Issues

Finally, the last big problem that can occur with low carb diets are adherence issues. Unless you're someone who just doesn't crave carbohydrates at all, there's going to be a point where cravings hit and it's all you can do to keep yourself away from the bread basket (or box of crackers, cereal, pasta – whatever your preference happens to be).

If you can't fight these cravings, very often they will lead to an 'all out binge' where you take in a massive amount of calories at once, really doing yourself in as far as overall results are concerned.

So there you have the primary issues that low carb diets can present. They definitely can be a good way to set up a diet, but very often it's a wiser decision to use some of the principles from them and tweak them to your own needs and preferences. By doing so you create the best diet for yourself and that's what is really going to get you the results you're after.

If you are comfortable and happy with your diet then you're going to stick with it and that, at the end of the day is the single biggest contributor to progress.

What I suggest instead is focusing on a diet plan that chooses the *right* types of carbohydrates at the right time and in the right quantities. If you do that, you're golden.

Now let's have a look at what the 'right type' of carbohydrates consists of.

There are four main types of carbohydrates that you should know about, starchy complex carbohydrates (SCC), fruit complex carbohydrates (FCC), vegetable complex carbohydrates (VCC), and simple carbohydrates (SC).

Each of these will react slightly differently in the body so it's vital that you learn these differences so you can select appropriately and add them to your diet when needed. Let's go over each one individually.

Starchy Complex Carbohydrates

The very first form of carbohydrates to know about is starchy complex carbohydrates. These are going to be the ones that break down quite slowly in the body, releasing a steady stream of glucose into the blood over time.

Since they are composed of complex structures of glucose molecules, they will not go to the liver like fructose would (as we discussed earlier) but instead will be taken up into the blood and then directed into the muscle cells, used for energy, or, in times of high calorie intakes, converted to body fat.

Since they do have that low impact on blood sugar levels however, you'll find that they don't leave you feeling nearly as hungry as quickly as some of the other forms of carbohydrates do.

The typical foods that represent SCC include:

- Sweet potatoes**
- Brown rice**
- Whole wheat pasta
- Whole grain bread
- Whole grain/bran cereals
- Beans* **
- Legumes* **
- Quinoa* **
- Barley
- Buckwheat**
- Whole wheat wraps/tortillas
- Cornmeal**
- Rice Flour**
- Millet**

*Denotes higher protein options for vegetarians
**Denotes gluten-free options

Eating moderate amounts of these throughout the day will help to maintain energy levels and keep your hunger levels in check. You do have to be careful not to overdo them however as they do contain more calories and this can add up quickly. Take in two cups of brown rice for instance and even though it is technically considered a healthy food, you've still just consumed 400 calories.

Fruit Complex Carbohydrates

The next type of carb source is fruit complex carbohydrates. Fruit often gets a bad rap by those who are dieting since they feel it is too high in 'sugar', but recall how we talked about the fact that half of the carbohydrates found in fruit are actually fructose, which doesn't spike insulin levels like pure sugar would.

Fruit actually breaks down slightly lower in the body due to the fiber content it contains therefore you won't see a sharp spike in blood glucose either. What's more is that many people find fruit to be highly satiating on a lower carbohydrate plan, therefore adding one to two pieces per day can be a very good method for beating the hunger bug.

The important thing to remember here is just to ensure that you maintain your desired calorie intake. Fruits do contain more calories than vegetables do, so they aren't a 'free for all' when it comes to your diet. You must make sure that you are still keeping track of how many you're eating and scheduling them into your diet.

The other thing to keep in mind with the fruit intake is that you will want to avoid fruit immediately after the workout period. At this point you want to maximize the amount of muscle glycogen that gets into the muscle tissues and since fruit is only half glucose, the additional fructose that's found in it will do nothing for improving your post-workout replenishment and recovery.

Save the fruit for a later time in the day and then choose starchy complex carbohydrates or simple carbohydrates (which we'll discuss shortly) instead.

Fruit complex carbohydrates include all varieties of fruit including:

- Apples
- Bananas
- Oranges
- Peaches
- Nectarines
- Grapes
- Strawberries
- Blueberries
- Raspberries
- Blackberries
- Pineapple (note much higher in sugar than the other varieties)
- Dates (also much higher in sugar than the other varieties)
- Melons

Fruits will vary slightly in their calorie content so it's worth checking out for your reference but in most instances, you're looking at about 60-90 calories per whole fruit or 50-80 calories per cup.

**Note that all fruits are gluten free.

Vegetable Complex Carbohydrates

Now we come to vegetable complex carbohydrates. These are going to be one of the best forms of carbohydrates for the dieter to eat because they provide a wealth of different nutrients, pack a very powerful fiber punch, and are so incredibly low in calories that you can virtually eat as many as you want without it impacting your total calorie intake.

If there is such a thing as 'free foods' on a diet plan, vegetables would be it.

One important thing to note with vegetables though is that there are a few that would be considered SCC instead due to their higher sugar content.

These are carrots, peas, corn, and turnips. While you certainly can add these to your diet since they are filled with plenty of good nutrients, you need to be more careful about how much you add as they will have a larger impact on blood sugar levels and your overall calorie intake.

The few carbohydrates that VCC do contain release very slowly in the body due to their high fiber content and are one food that will provide a high feeling of fullness immediately after the meal. Try and fill your plate at least half full with vegetables at each meal you eat and if you can incorporate a few into your snack choices as well, all the better.

As long as you are making sure to prepare your vegetables without any heavy sauces or other calorie or high fat ingredients then you can virtually eat as many of them as you like while maintaining your diet plan.

Such vegetable choices include:

- Broccoli
- Cauliflower
- Mushrooms
- Onions
- Peppers
- Cabbage
- Lettuce (romaine, head, leaf, etc)
- Asparagus
- Spinach*
- Bean sprouts
- Seaweed*
- and so on….

*Denotes higher protein options for vegetarians
**All vegetables are gluten free

Don't ever feel restricted with your vegetable intake because these are here to help you progress through your diet and see the best results possible from your hard efforts.

Simple Carbohydrates

Finally the last type of carbohydrates that you must make yourself aware of are the simple carbohydrates. These carbohydrates are the main ones that you'll be working to eliminate from your diet entirely as they are the ones that will cause quick blood sugar spikes followed by drops and promote you to eat more and more food.

If you're not watching carefully you can easily overcome a vast number of calories and really put a dent in your weight loss. For many people simply eliminating these from their diet plan is enough to get them to start seeing the fat loss they're after so that's something that you will definitely want to take into account. It's one simple change but can have a world of difference.

Simple carbohydrates are the ones that also put you at a greater risk of developing diseases such as diabetes because they place a lot more stress on the body due to the high insulin release they cause. Over time this really wears on you and eventually you may find that your body simply does not respond to insulin like it used to, hence more and more needs to be pumped out in order to control the carbohydrate intake. Do this often enough for a long period of time and eventually you may just find yourself requiring insulin in order to keep up with the blood sugar increase and maintain control.

Obviously this is a situation you want to avoid, and by limiting the amount of SC in your diet you will do so effectively.

Now, the one exception to this rule – the one time when you actually may want to include SC in your diet is right before and after your workout period. At this point in time it's actually ideal to get a big blood sugar spike followed by a crash since this is going to allow you to replenish the muscle glycogen levels the fastest since the insulin released will drive them into the cells of the body.

You still must ensure to count these calories into your daily diet but during this point, some simple carbs is ideal. If you find you suffer from very sensitive blood sugar levels then you may want to consider mixing together some simple carbohydrates along with some starchy carbohydrates for best results.

So what do simple carbohydrates consist of?

Generally speaking the following foods will fall into this category:

- Cakes
- Cookies
- Candy
- Soda
- Snack crackers
- Snack/energy bars
- Fruit bars
- Fruit beverages
- Chips
- White flour baked goods
- White rice
- White bread and bread products
- Sugary cereals
- Rice chips
- Chocolate/candy bars

Essentially, anything that doesn't come from the ground or looks like it's been through some form of processing will fall into the simple carbs category.

One thing that you should keep in mind here though is that immediately after the workout your body is actually hungry for a bit of sugar. Since the muscle glycogen has just been depleted, you could actually take in a few simple carbs and they'll do your body good.

Since at this point they'll move directly into the muscle cells to resaturate the muscle glycogen, this will improve your overall recovery.

So keeping this in mind, if you do decide that you are craving a food that is higher in sugar content, placing it immediately after your workout is a wise move.

This doesn't mean you have free reign to go off eating junk food around every workout session, but all I'm saying is that if you are having a seriously strong craving, by being smart with when you do decide to give in you can actually have that food work in your favour rather than against you.

Dairy products also have some simple carbohydrates in them, however these carbohydrates are referred to as 'lactose' and aren't quite the concern that straight glucose is.

Some people will experience issues digesting this form of carbohydrates however (when they suffer from lactose intolerance) so that's something that you'll want to keep in mind.

If you find that you're always bloated or have very bad gas after consuming dairy products, it may be worth your while to avoid them for a short period of time and see if that issue improves itself.

Dairy products also contain some protein as well so typically these will not have the negative influence on the blood sugar level that pure glucose will as the protein helps to slow the overall rate of digestion.

So there you have the basic background information on the different types of carbohydrates there are and how these are going to react in your body.

If you do want to feel and look your best, making sure that you place them properly in your diet is going to be vital.

Now let's talk a little bit about how many carbohydrates to eat and carb timing for best results.

How Many Carbohydrates To Consume

We've already given you a recommend guideline for how much protein you should be consuming on a daily basis, next comes factoring in how many carbohydrates you should eat.

Your carbohydrate intake will be very dependant on your overall activity levels and how quickly you want to experience fat loss because the more active you are, the more carbohydrates you will require and likewise, the faster you want to lose body fat, the lower you should be taking those carbohydrates.

As a general rule, those who are doing more strength training work should add more carbohydrates to their diets, especially around those workout sessions since the body is really going to need them at that point.

For most people, a good starting point for their carbohydrate intake when aiming to lose body fat will be around 1-1.5 grams per pound of body weight. For those who are much more active throughout the day you may be able to bring this up to 2 grams per pound but make note that you still must be maintaining the overall calorie balance.

Remember that carbohydrates contain four calories per gram, so if you weigh 150 pounds and are taking in 2 grams per pound, that means 300 grams per day or 1200 calories worth.

Those who are much less active or who want to experience fat loss at a much faster pace may decide to bring their overall carbohydrate intake lower than the one gram per pound per day mark, but do keep in mind that if you bring it below 100 grams per day, the body may start fighting you on this as this is the number of carbohydrates needed in order for the brain to function optimally.

Keep in mind too that you definitely can have some higher carb days in your weekly schedule and then some lower carb days in the plan as well to coincide on days that you are more active. This is a great way to set-up the overall design since then you will supply more energy in times of need but cut back when you don't.

Timing Your Carbohydrate Intake

One thing that is very smart to do as you go about setting up your diet is timing your carbohydrate intake properly. This means placing more of the complex carbohydrates (or SC if you're eating them pre/post workout) earlier on in the day when you are more active and around the workout period and then focusing on just having vegetable carbohydrates as well as fruit carbohydrates later on in the day with the other meals.

Since you won't need quite as much energy later on while you're just lounging around, this is ideal for setting up your diet.

So your day may look something like this:

Breakfast: SCC + Protein + Fat

Snack: VCC or FCC + Protein

Lunch: VCC + Protein + Fat

Pre-Workout Snack: FCC + Protein

Post-Workout Snack: SCC + Protein

Dinner: Protein + Fat + VCC

Before Bed Snack: Protein + Fat + VCC

SCC = Stachy Complex Carbohydrate

FCC = Fruit Complex Carbohydrate

VCC = Vegetable Complex Carbohydrate

As you work with your trainer, they may adjust your meal plan slightly based on your goals to make sure that you're burning a maximum amount of body fat.

This gives you a very nice distribution of the three main macronutrients: proteins, carbohydrates, and fats, while spreading your calorie intake out throughout the day for greater overall satiety.

How you choose to place the carbohydrates in your diet will always be up to you but by keeping these points in mind, you should find that your energy levels are more stable, you recover faster from your workouts, and you begin looking much, much leaner than you were before.

Now let's shift our focus over to the fat component of your diet.

CHAPTER 11:
ALL ABOUT FATS

Now that we've discussed both proteins and carbohydrates, it's time to look at the third macronutrient that you should be taking into account, dietary fats. Dietary fats are often avoided by many dieters because they contain over twice as many calories per gram (9, while, as mentioned proteins and carbohydrates only contain 4) and will really drive that total calorie intake up higher if you aren't watching yourself.

When eaten in moderation though fats should be a part of a healthy diet because they do offer so many vital nutrients that you need. They're going to help keep your hair and skin looking healthy and will help ensure that all the reproduction organs stay functioning optimally (this is especially important if you're a woman).

In short, eliminating all the fats from your diet would be a very big mistake and could cost you significantly in the long term results you see on both your body composition and your health.

Another nice thing about dietary fats is that they are digested very slowly by the body so you will find that you feel much fuller for a longer period of time by consuming them.

Having a meal consisting of protein and healthy fats can keep you satisfied for hours, while if you would have eaten the same meal consisting of protein and carbohydrates, you may be back in the cupboard looking for more a short hour later.

Usually all it takes to boost up the overall level of satiety you feel from dietary fats is around 5-7 grams per meal, so this would account for about 35-65 calories total – hardly anything when put in the context of your total calorie intake.

If you keep it to around this amount for all of your meals you shouldn't find it a problem in terms of maintaining your fat loss calorie balance.

There's no real reason to take fat over and above this amount per meal unless you are using a lower carb/higher fat approach to your diet or have a higher calorie intake and have calories to fill.

Usually though, assuming you aren't carbohydrate sensitive, you'd be slightly better off increasing the amount of carbohydrates around the workout period if you have calories to fill since this ensures your muscle glycogen levels are always saturated and that you are not experiencing the negative issues from leptin that were described on page 76.

Moving on, another vital thing that you must know about your dietary fat intake is that not all fats are created equally. You have some fats that will do nothing but hinder your overall health and body composition while there are other fats that will help to promote it.

In order to get the most from your diet you'll want to be sure to be taking in plenty of the healthy fats, while limiting the unhealthy varieties.

Let's take a look at the fats a little more closely.

Monounsaturated and Polyunsaturated Fats

The first variety of fats that you'll want to include in your diet are monounsaturated and polyunsaturated fats. These are known to be the 'healthy' fats to consume and are going to provide benefits such as helping you maintain healthy blood cholesterol levels, helping to ward off various diseases, helping to ensure that the skin, organs, and hair stay healthy, and for helping to provide a long term energy source when in need.

Foods that will provide you with sources of monounsaturated and polyunsaturated fat include:

- Olive oil
- Peanut oil
- Canola oil
- Safflower oil
- Corn oil
- Sunflower oil
- Soy oil
- Cottonseed oil
- Nuts
- Natural nut butters
- Seeds

Other foods that you consume in your diet may also provide sources of unsaturated fat in smaller varieties but since they often don't really account for much at all are not included in this list.

Essential Fatty Acids

The next type of dietary fat has received quite a bit of attention lately and for good reason – the health benefits it provides are very diverse and vital.

Essentially fatty acids, sometimes referred to as omega-3 fatty acids are going to really go a long way towards promoting a healthy heart and will also help to counteract issues such as insulin resistance.

Essential fatty acids can also promote the burning of body fat for fuel purposes so they are very critical when trying to get leaner and reach your goal body weight.

Foods that are rich in essential fatty acids that you should be including in your diet are:

- Fatty cold water fish (salmon, mackerel, herring)
- Flaxseeds
- Flaxseed oil
- Walnuts
- Fish oil caps

It's very important that you're making sure to take in some essential fatty acids throughout the week as if you don't eat a lot of fatty fish this is one nutrient that many people do miss out on.

Usually the simplest way to remedy this problem is to rely on an essential fatty acid supplement such as fish oil caps that you can easily take throughout the day with your meals.

Ideally if you are going to use this manner to meet your needs you would want to aim for about 3-6 grams of essential fatty acids daily.

Saturated Fats

The next type of fat we come to are the saturated fats and these are a lot more harmful to the body. Saturated fats are the ones that will clog your arteries and increase your chances of heart disease, diabetes, or even stroke.

Those who have diets that are very high in saturated fat often find that their cholesterol levels are very much in favour of a negative profile and that in itself can quickly put your health in jeopardy.

Usually it's virtually impossible to eliminate all saturated fat from the diet since it is commonly found in many food sources that you should be eating to maintain good health, however, if you are choosing the right types of foods then it can be kept to a relatively low minimum.

Ideally you should take in somewhere between 5-15% of your total fat content from saturated fats which will be best for optimum health as well as for helping you to maintain ideal levels of sex hormones.

Whenever you drop the saturated fat too low in the diet you do risk suffering from problems with the sex hormones (testosterone, estrogen, and progesterone), so for that reason you shouldn't completely eliminate it entirely at any point.

The foods where saturated fat is most commonly found include:

- Fatty sources of meat (beef, dark meat chicken, etc)
- Sausage
- High fat dairy products
- Eggs
- Lard
- Butter
- Coconut oil
- Palm oil
- Processed and snack foods
- Baked goods

Trans Fats

Finally the last source of fat that you will want to ensure that you're especially careful about are trans fats. These fats are by far the most harmful to humans and do not occur by nature alone.

Rather, they are a type of dietary fat that has come to be through our own processing and manufacturing and will wreak havoc on the body.

Trans fats occur whenever a regular fat molecule goes through a process of hydrogenation, where an additional hydrogen molecule is added to the structure.

Trans fats are more solid by nature than oil is; meaning that they are less likely to spoil, which is a big reason why you'll usually find this fat mostly on the shelves lining the supermarket. These have a very long shelf-life and have a non-greasy feel to them so many food manufacturers prefer using them in their products.

Any time you see the term 'partially hydrogenated vegetable oil'; you know right there that that product contains trans fats. Immediately you should be placing it back onto the shelf as it's not going to be doing you any health favours whatsoever.

There are no specific requirements for trans fats in the diet and it is actually recommended that you avoid these entirely.

The most common sources of trans fats include:

- Crackers
- Cookies
- Cakes
- Pastries
- Snack bars
- French fries
- Donuts
- Shortenings
- Margarines (in some cases)
- Fast food

The very important thing to remember when it comes to trans fats is that by law right now a food company does not have to list trans fats on their nutritional panel if the product contains less than 0.5 grams per serving.

But, if you were to eat five or six of these foods each day, this can add up and you could be taking in 3-5 grams on a daily basis. This may not seem like all that much fat but when it comes to trans fats, any fat is too much.

Really do your best to scan the ingredient listings instead and any time you see the word 'hydrogenated' in the listings, avoid it at all costs.

So there you have some info on the main types of fats that are found in the foods you eat.

It's important to understand how to set up the fat intake in your diet. Ideally you want to be mixing together your healthy fat intake with your protein based meals that come later on in the day when you're less active. This way, you can maintain a good calorie intake for that meal in particular and will find that your hunger levels stay under control far better.

The one thing that you must do though is avoid fat right before and after the workout period because taking it in at this time is only going to slow the digestion process and that can result in you feeling weighed down and lethargic.

In addition to that, since the point during the post workout period is to get the nutrients into the muscle cells as fast as possible, having a high dietary fat intake is going to go directly against achieving that goal.

Setting Your Dietary Fat Intake

When it comes to setting your dietary fat intake, this is going to largely depend on how many calories you're taking in on your fat loss diet as well as how many carbohydrates you decided to add into your diet.

Since protein is set at a certain amount, you're going to find an inverse relationship with carbohydrates and dietary fat where the more carbs you take in, the fewer total fat you'll consume.

Those who choose to use a higher carb approach to their diet will take in fewer grams of fat over the course of the day while those who choose to use a higher fat diet will take in more.

Remember that protein and carbs each contain four calories per gram so to get how much total fat you should be aiming for you'll simply subtract your total carb and protein values from your total calorie target and divide by nine to get grams.

Distribute this fat intake over the meals during the point of the day when you're less active and you'll be right on track.

This now concludes our discussion of coming up with your diet plan. Keep all of this advice in mind and set out your own plan tailored to your own individual needs and preferences.

Included in this book are a variety of meal plans that you can feel free to use or if you'd like, come up with some of your own. The important thing is just making sure you do have a plan as that is what will keep you on track.

In the next section, we'll go over exactly how to do this.

CHAPTER 12:
FORMING YOUR FAMILY MEAL PLAN

For many of you, one of the challenges of coming up with a diet that you're going to stick with is making sure that you create meals that your family will enjoy.

If you're a parent and have young children at home, there's no question that often they will turn their nose up at some of the 'healthier' foods that you may decide to serve.

The key here is discovering new and innovative methods of improving the taste of healthy dishes so that they satisfy both your and their nutrient requirements while also pleasing the taste buds.

Fortunately, with some simple and easy to implement tricks, this is more than possible.

That's why I've put together an easy to follow family meal plan that will satisfy almost all taste preferences.

Using the foods from our food lists you're going to get high quality nutrition in easy to prepare meals that will make sure you can eat healthy while you're on the run.

*Note that I've included both workout and non-workout days in the meal plan. If your workout days happen to fall on different days than what's shown below, simply re-arrange the plans as such. The only difference will be the afternoon pre/post workout meals versus the afternoon snack.

MONDAY:

Meal	Food
Breakfast	½ cup oatmeal (dry measurement)
	6 egg whites
	1 tbsp natural almond butter
Snack	1 small apple
	½ cup low-fat cottage cheese
Lunch	3 oz chicken
	2 cups spinach leaves
	Grape tomatoes, red onions, and sliced red peppers
	1 tbsp olive oil dressing
Pre-Workout	1 orange
	1 scoop whey protein powder
Post-Workout	2 slices Ezekiel bread with no sugar added jam
	1 scoop whey protein powder
Dinner	3 oz lean steak
	2 cups steamed broccoli
	15 almonds
Before Bed Snack (If hungry and no later than 1 hr before bed)	½ cup Liberte Greek Yogurt
	20 pistachios

TUESDAY:

Meal	Food
Breakfast	1 cup bran cereal
	1 cup skim milk (lactose free)
	2 tbsp flaxseeds
Snack	10 carrot sticks
	1 small can of tuna, drained
	Dijon Mustard
Lunch	3 oz low-sodium deli meat
	2 cups mixed greens
	1 tbsp olive oil vinaigrette
	Any other vegetables desired
Snack	3 oz chicken breast
	½ cup grapes
Dinner	3 oz salmon
	5 spears steamed asparagus
	1 tbsp olive oil
Before Bed Snack (If hungry and no later than 1 hr before bed)	½ cup low-fat cottage cheese
	1 tbsp natural almond butter

WEDNESDAY:

Meal	Food
Breakfast	¼ cup oatmeal (dry measurement)
	4 egg whites
	½ scoop whey protein powder
	½ cup sliced strawberries
Snack	½ cup Liberte Greek Yogurt
	½ cup blueberries
Lunch	3 oz turkey
	2 cups steamed cauliflower and broccoli
	15 almonds
Pre-Workout	1 scoop whey protein powder
	½ cup grapes
Post-Workout	1 scoop whey protein powder
	1 cup Kashi Go Lean cereal
Dinner	4 oz cod fish
	2 cups stir-fried mixed vegetables
	1 tbsp olive oil
Before Bed Snack (If hungry and no later than 1 hr before bed)	3 oz chicken breast
	10 celery sticks
	10 almonds

THURSDAY:

Meal	Food
Breakfast	1 Ezekiel 4:9 whole grain English muffin 6 egg whites 2 slices tomato 1 oz 4% Allegro lactose free cheese
Snack	1 scoop whey protein powder 1 apple
Lunch	1 small can of tuna, drained 2 cups spinach 6 grape tomatoes 1 tbsp olive oil dressing
Snack	1 serving Quick and Easy anytime super shake or bar
Dinner	4 oz salmon 2 cups steamed bok choy 1 tbsp olive oil
Before Bed Snack (If hungry and no later than 1 hr before bed)	½ cup Liberte Greek Yogurt 1 tbsp natural almond butter

FRIDAY:

Meal	Food
Breakfast	6 egg whites
	2 tbsp salsa (No sugar added)
	1 orange
	1 tbsp olive oil
Snack	½ cup Liberte Greek Yogurt
	½ cup blueberries
Lunch	3 oz chicken breast
	1 cup steamed broccoli
	15 almonds
Pre-Workout	1 scoop whey protein powder
	1 apple
Post-Workout	1 scoop whey protein powder
	1 slice Ezekiel bread with no sugar added jam
Dinner	4 oz lean beef
	5 spears grilled asparagus
	1 tbsp olive oil
Before Bed Snack (If hungry and no later than 1 hr before bed)	1 hard boiled egg
	Raw vegetables if desired

SATURDAY:

Meal	Food
Breakfast	3 oz lean ham meat 1 small sweet potato 1 tbsp olive oil
Snack	1 serving Quick and Easy anytime super shake or bar
Lunch	3 oz turkey 2 cups steamed cauliflower 2 tbsp flaxseeds or 1 tbsp flaxseed oil
Snack	1 small can tuna, drained Sliced mushrooms and peppers 2 tbsp salsa (No sugar added)
Dinner	4 oz cod fish 5 spears steamed asparagus Lemon juice 1 tbsp olive oil
Before Bed Snack (If hungry and no later than 1 hr before bed)	½ cup low-fat cottage cheese 1 tbsp almond butter

SUNDAY:

Meal	Food
Breakfast	¼ cup oatmeal (dry measurement)
	6 egg whites
	Chopped vegetables
	1 tbsp olive oil
Snack	½ cup Liberte Greek Yogurt
	½ cup blackberries
Lunch	3 oz low-sodium chicken breast deli meat
	3-4 large lettuce leaves (used as a 'wrap' for meat)
	Sliced cucumbers and tomatoes
	2 oz 4% Allegro lactose free cheese
Snack	1 glass skim milk (lactose free)
	1 peach
Dinner	3 oz pork tenderloin
	2 cups green beans
	1 tbsp olive oil
	Spices as desired
Before Bed Snack (If hungry and no later than 1 hr before bed)	½ cup Liberte Greek Yogurt
	10 almonds

CHAPTER 13:
FORMING YOUR VEGETARIAN MEAL PLAN

If you're someone who prefers the vegetarian lifestyle, this does not mean that you can't reach your fitness goals. While it may be a little more challenging to get in enough of the lean protein that you need, as long as you do some proper planning and take the time to consider all the sources that you do have available to you, it's more than possible.

*Note that for this diet we assumed you are eating dairy products and eggs, however if you do not wish to include these in your diet then you'll simply want to opt for some other vegetarian protein sources such as soy or tofu.

MONDAY:

Meal	Food
Breakfast	½ cup oatmeal (dry measurement)
	6 egg whites
	1 tbsp natural peanut butter
Snack	1 small apple
	½ cup low-fat cottage cheese
Lunch	3 oz tofu
	2 cups spinach leaves
	Grape tomatoes, red onions, and sliced red peppers
	1 tbsp olive oil dressing
Pre-Workout	1 pear
	1 scoop whey protein powder
Post-Workout	2 slices Ezekiel bread with no sugar added jam
	1 scoop whey protein powder
Dinner	100 grams tempeh
	2 cups steamed broccoli
	15 almonds
Before Bed Snack (If hungry and no later than 1 hr before bed)	½ cup Liberte Greek Yogurt
	20 pistachios

TUESDAY:

Meal	Food
Breakfast	1 cup bran cereal
	1 cup low-fat soy milk original/natural
	2 tbsp flaxseeds
Snack	10 baby carrot sticks
	5 tbsp hummus
	2 oz Allegro 4% lactose free cheese
Lunch	3 oz Tofu
	2 cups mixed greens
	1 tbsp olive oil vinaigrette
	Any other vegetables desired
Snack	1 veggie burger (without the bun)
	½ cup grapes
Dinner	3 oz ground soy mixed with 1 egg white and made into a patty
	5 spears steamed asparagus
	1 tbsp olive oil
Before Bed Snack (If hungry and no later than 1 hr before bed)	½ cup low-fat cottage cheese
	1 tbsp natural peanut butter

WEDNESDAY:

Meal	Food
Breakfast	¼ cup oatmeal (dry measurement)
	4 egg whites
	½ scoop whey protein powder
	½ cup sliced strawberries
Snack	½ cup Liberte Greek Yogurt
	1 peach
Lunch	2 veggie dogs
	2 cups steamed cauliflower and broccoli
	15 almonds
Pre-Workout	1 scoop whey protein powder
	½ cup grapes
Post-Workout	1 scoop whey protein powder
	1 cup Kashi Go Lean cereal
Dinner	100 grams Tempeh
	2 cups stir-fried mixed vegetables
	1 tbsp olive oil
Before Bed Snack (If hungry and no later than 1 hr before bed)	1 cup Liberte Greek Yogurt
	10 celery sticks
	10 almonds

THURSDAY:

Meal	Food
Breakfast	1 Ezekiel 4:9 whole grain English muffin
	6 egg whites
	2 slices tomato
	1 oz 4% Allegro lactose free cheese
Snack	1 scoop whey protein powder
	1 apple
Lunch	1 veggie burger crumbled over salad
	2 cups spinach
	Grape tomatoes
	1 tbsp olive oil dressing
Snack	1 serving Quick and Easy anytime super shake or bar
Dinner	100 grams Tofu
	2 cups steamed bok choy
	1 tbsp olive oil
Before Bed Snack (If hungry and no later than 1 hr before bed)	½ cup Liberte Greek Yogurt
	1 tbsp natural peanut butter

FRIDAY:

Meal	Food
Breakfast	6 egg whites 2 tbsp salsa (No sugar added) 1 orange 1 tbsp olive oil
Snack	½ cup Liberte Greek Yogurt ½ cup blueberries
Lunch	3 oz ground soy mixed with 1 egg white and made into a patty 1 cup steamed broccoli 15 almonds
Pre-Workout	1 scoop whey protein powder 1 grapefruit
Post-Workout	1 scoop whey protein powder 1 slice Ezekiel bread with no sugar added jam
Dinner	100 grams Tempeh 5 spears grilled asparagus 1 tbsp olive oil
Before Bed Snack (If hungry and no later than 1 hr before bed)	1 hard boiled egg Raw vegetables if desired

SATURDAY:

Meal	Food
Breakfast	2 soy sausages 1 small sweet potato 1 tbsp olive oil
Snack	1 serving Quick and Easy anytime super shake or bar
Lunch	1 veggie burger 2 cups steamed cauliflower 2 tbsp flaxseeds or 1 tbsp flaxseed oil
Snack	½ cup low-fat cottage cheese ½ cup grapes
Dinner	100 grams tofu 5 spears steamed asparagus Lemon juice 1 tbsp olive oil
Before Bed Snack (If hungry and no later than 1 hr before bed)	½ cup low-fat cottage cheese 1 tbsp almond butter

SUNDAY:

Meal	Food
Breakfast	¼ cup oatmeal (dry measurement)
	4 slices soy bacon
	1 tbsp olive oil
Snack	½ cup Liberte Greek Yogurt
	½ cup blackberries
Lunch	3 oz Tofu
	3-4 large lettuce leaves (used as a 'wrap' for meat)
	Sliced cucumbers and tomatoes
	2 oz 4% Allegro lactose free cheese
Snack	1 glass low-fat soy milk original/natural
	1 apple
Dinner	3 oz ground soy mixed with 1 egg white and made into a patty
	2 cups green beans
	1 tbsp olive oil
	Spices as desired
Before Bed Snack (If hungry and no later than 1 hr before bed)	½ cup Librete Greek Yogurt
	10 almonds

CHAPTER 14:
FORMING YOUR GLUTEN-FREE MEAL PLAN

Dealing with a gluten intolerance can be a frustrating thing but if you do make the effort to make sure you're eating right and are not including gluten in your everyday diet, you're going to find that the payoff is profound.

You'll have more energy, you won't feel sick to your stomach any longer, and you'll easily be able to lose the weight that's been troubling you for all these years.

MONDAY:

Meal	Food
Breakfast	1 banana
	1 cup berries
	6 egg whites
	1 tbsp natural peanut butter
Snack	1 small apple
	½ cup low-fat cottage cheese
Lunch	3 oz chicken
	2 cups spinach leaves
	Grape tomatoes, red onions, and sliced red peppers
	1 tbsp olive oil mixed with balsamic vinegar
Pre-Workout	1 peach
	1 scoop whey protein powder
Post-Workout	1 cup quinoa
	1 scoop whey protein powder
Dinner	3 oz lean steak
	2 cups steamed broccoli
	15 almonds
Before Bed Snack (If hungry and no later than 1 hr before bed)	½ cup Liberte Greek Yogurt
	20 pistachios

TUESDAY:

Meal	Food
Breakfast	1 cup brown rice
	1 cup skim milk (lactose free)
	1 tsp cinnamon
	1 tsp honey or sweetener
	2 tbsp flaxseeds
Snack	10 carrot sticks
	1 small can tuna, drained
	2 tbsp salsa (No sugar added)
Lunch	3 oz low-sodium deli meat
	2 cups mixed greens
	1 tbsp olive oil and balsamic vinegar
	Any other vegetables desired
Snack	3 oz chicken breast
	½ cup grapes
Dinner	3 oz salmon
	5 spears steamed asparagus
	1 tbsp olive oil
Before Bed Snack (If hungry and no later than 1 hr before bed)	½ cup low-fat cottage cheese
	1 tbsp natural peanut butter

WEDNESDAY:

Meal	Food
Breakfast	4 egg whites + 1 whole egg
	½ scoop whey protein powder
	½ cup sliced strawberries
	½ cup blueberries
Snack	½ cup Liberte Greek Yogurt
	1 peach
Lunch	3 oz turkey
	2 cups steamed cauliflower and broccoli
	15 almonds
Pre-Workout	1 scoop whey protein powder
	½ cup grapes
Post-Workout	1 scoop whey protein powder
	1 large sweet potato baked with cinnamon and a touch of honey
Dinner	4 oz cod fish
	2 cups stir-fried mixed vegetables
	1 tbsp olive oil
Before Bed Snack (If hungry and no later than 1 hr before bed)	3 oz chicken breast
	10 celery sticks
	10 almonds

THURSDAY:

Meal	Food
Breakfast	6 egg whites
	2 slices tomato
	1 oz 4% Allegro lactose free cheese
	1 banana
Snack	1 scoop whey protein powder
	1 apple
Lunch	1 small can of tuna, drained
	2 cups spinach
	Grape tomatoes
	1 tbsp olive oil mixed with balsamic vinegar
Snack	1 serving Quick and Easy anytime super shake or bar
Dinner	4 oz salmon
	2 cups steamed bok choy
	1 tbsp olive oil
Before Bed Snack (If hungry and no later than 1 hr before bed)	½ cup Liberte Greek Yogurt
	1 tbsp natural peanut butter

FRIDAY:

Meal	Food
Breakfast	6 egg whites
	2 tbsp salsa (No sugar added)
	1 orange
	1 tbsp olive oil
Snack	½ cup Liberte Greek Yogurt
	½ cup blueberries
Lunch	3 oz chicken breast
	1 cup steamed broccoli
	15 almonds
Pre-Workout	1 scoop whey protein powder
	1 grapefruit
Post-Workout	1 scoop whey protein powder
	1 cup quinoa
Dinner	4 oz lean beef
	5 spears grilled asparagus
	1 tbsp olive oil
Before Bed Snack (If hungry and no later than 1 hr before bed)	1 hard boiled egg
	Raw vegetables if desired

SATURDAY:

Meal	Food
Breakfast	3 oz lean ham meat 1 small sweet potato 1 tbsp olive oil
Snack	1 serving Quick and Easy anytime super shake or bar
Lunch	3 oz turkey 2 cups steamed cauliflower 2 tbsp flaxseeds or 1 tbsp flaxseed oil
Snack	1 small can tuna, drained Sliced mushrooms and peppers
Dinner	4 oz cod fish 5 spears steamed asparagus Lemon juice 1 tbsp olive oil
Before Bed Snack (If hungry and no later than 1 hr before bed)	½ cup low-fat cottage cheese 1 tbsp almond butter

SUNDAY:

Meal	Food
Breakfast	6 egg whites Chopped vegetables 1 tbsp olive oil 2 cups melon, chopped
Snack	½ cup Liberte Greek Yogurt ½ cup blackberries
Lunch	3 oz low-sodium chicken breast deli meat 3-4 large lettuce leaves (used as a 'wrap' for meat) Sliced cucumbers and tomatoes 2 oz 4% Allegro lactose free cheese
Snack	1 glass skim milk (lactose free) 1 peach
Dinner	3 oz pork tenderloin 2 cups green beans 1 tbsp olive oil Spices as desired
Before Bed Snack (If hungry and no later than 1 hr before bed)	½ low-fat cottage cheese 10 almonds

CHAPTER 15:
FORMING YOUR GET RIPPED MEAL PLAN

When you need to get lean in a hurry, it's going to be time to really step up your diet and get strict with yourself. That's precisely what this plan is designed to do. You definitely will find that it keeps you on your toes and restricts some food that you normally would eat, but the payoff will be a whole new level of leanness that you've never experienced before.

The protein in this diet is very high to ensure that you aren't at risk for losing muscle mass and the carbohydrates are kept lower. Fat is included with most of your meals to help keep hunger down and energy levels higher.

Try this diet plan for two to three weeks and you can be guaranteed that you'll notice a difference in how you look.

MONDAY:

Meal	Food
Breakfast	6 egg whites
	Diced vegetables
	1 tsp olive oil
Snack	1 small can Tuna, drained
	Chopped celery
	2 tbsp salsa (No sugar added)
Lunch	3 oz chicken breast
	5 spears steamed asparagus
	Lemon juice
Pre-Workout	1 scoop whey protein powder
	1 cup strawberries
Post-Workout	1 scoop whey protein powder
	¼ cup oatmeal (dry measurement)
Dinner	3 oz tilapia
	2 cups steamed broccoli
	10 almonds
Before Bed Snack (If hungry and no later than 1 hr before bed)	½ cup low-fat cottage cheese

TUESDAY:

Meal	Food
Breakfast	6 egg whites
	Diced vegetables
	1 tsp olive oil
Snack	3 oz Tilapia
	½ cucumber sliced
	2 tbsp salsa (No sugar added)
Lunch	3 oz chicken breast
	2 cups steamed broccoli
	Garlic or any other spice desired
Snack	2 hard boiled Omega-3 egg (No yolk)
	1 cup celery and carrot sticks
Dinner	3 oz extra lean sirloin steak
	5 spears steamed asparagus
	1 tbsp olive oil
Before Bed Snack (If hungry and no later than 1 hr before bed)	½ cup low-fat cottage cheese
	½ tbsp natural almond butter

WEDNESDAY:

Meal	Food
Breakfast	4 strips low fat or fat free turkey bacon
	Diced veggies
	Olive oil
Snack	1 orange
	1 small can of tuna, drained
Lunch	3 oz turkey meat
	2 cups stir-fried sliced vegetables
	1 tbsp olive oil
Pre-Workout	1 scoop whey protein powder
	1 pear
Post-Workout	1 scoop whey protein powder
	¼ cup oatmeal (dry measurement)
Dinner	4 oz Cod fish
	2 cups steamed bok choy
	Lemon juice
	10 almonds
Before Bed Snack (If hungry and no later than 1 hr before bed)	6 egg whites
	½ tbsp natural peanut butter

THURSDAY:

Meal	Food
Breakfast	6 egg whites
	Diced vegetables
	2 tbsp salsa (No sugar added)
	20 pistachios
Snack	½ cup low-fat cottage cheese
	½ cup sliced grapes
Lunch	3 oz extra lean ground turkey mixed with one egg white to form a patty
	2 cups spinach leaves
	1 tbsp olive oil and balsamic vinegar
Snack	10 grilled shrimp
Dinner	4 oz Tilapia
	5 spears steamed asparagus
	1 tbsp slivered almonds
Before Bed Snack (If hungry and no later than 1 hr before bed)	½ cup Liberte Greek Yogurt

FRIDAY:

Meal	Food
Breakfast	6 egg whites
	1 tbsp almond butter
	Coffee (No sugar)
Snack	1 small can of tuna, drained
	2 tbsp Salsa (No sugar added)
	Sliced red onions
Lunch	3 oz chicken breast
	Steamed broccoli and cauliflower
	10 almonds
Pre-Workout	1 scoop whey protein powder
	½ cup grapes
Post-Workout	1 scoop whey protein powder
	¼ cup oatmeal (dry measurement)
Dinner	3 oz lean sirloin steak
	Grilled red pepper
	2 cups spinach salad
	½ tbsp olive oil dressing
Before Bed Snack (If hungry and no later than 1 hr before bed)	½ cup low-fat cottage cheese

SATURDAY:

Meal	Food
Breakfast	4 strips low fat or fat free turkey bacon
	Stir-fried vegetables
	½ grapefruit
Snack	10 shrimp with lemon
Lunch	3 oz turkey breast
	2 cups mixed greens
	5 cherry tomatoes
	1 tbsp olive oil salad dressing
Snack	½ cup Liberte Greek Yogurt
Dinner	3 oz chicken breast
	Grilled mushrooms and peppers
	10 almonds
Before Bed Snack (If hungry and no later than 1 hr before bed)	6 egg whites
	½ tsp almond butter

SUNDAY:

Meal	Food
Breakfast	6 egg whites
	Diced vegetables
	2 tbsp Salsa (No added sugar)
Snack	1 small can of tuna, drained
	Balsamic vinegar
	Diced celery
Lunch	3 oz Venison meat
	2 cups steamed broccoli
	10 almonds
Snack	1 scoop whey protein powder
	½ cup mixed berries
Dinner	3 oz chicken breast
	5 spears steamed asparagus
	Lemon juice
	1 tbsp slivered almonds
Before Bed Snack (If hungry and no later than 1 hr before bed)	½ cup low-fat cottage cheese
	½ tbsp natural peanut butter

CHAPTER 16:
SUPPLEMENTS TO CONSIDER

Now that you have all of your meal plans all set out and ready to go, you might be wondering if there's any point in looking at some of the supplements that are available.

For many people, supplements are something that does tend to cause a bit of confusion because they've heard many mixed messages about them.

In some cases you may have heard that supplements are a great way to help meet your nutrient requirements and speed up the process of fat loss, but in other cases, you've heard that it's far better to get your nutrition from real food and that some of the fat loss products out there are only going to put your health at risk.

What's the consensus on this? Should you consider adding a supplement to your diet?

The thing you must keep in mind with this is what your primary reason for using the supplement is. If you're looking to use the supplement as a means to produce results for you (meaning you aren't paying all that much attention to your workout or diet plan, you're going to really struggle).

The biggest issue with supplementation is far too many individuals get very caught up with all of the hype surrounding them and start thinking that their supplement protocol can replace them from actually eating properly and performing hard workouts.

If this is your thinking pattern, you would be best off avoiding all supplements altogether since they will just be a distraction for you.

If, on the other hand you've already been working hard on your diet and fitness plan and have those both in place, then adding a supplement to the mix can be a good way to help further your progress along.

As long as you clearly understand what the limitations are of the supplement you're using and are using it appropriately, it shouldn't take away from the progress that you're making.

If this is in fact your case, how do you know which supplements to use?

Let's go over a few that are most helpful.

Multi-Vitamin

By far the most common supplement to use and one that you'll definitely want to include is a good quality multi-vitamin. This is going to be really important for ensuring that you aren't suffering from any nutrient deficiencies while you're on your reduced calorie diet and cutting back on your total food intake.

This doesn't mean you should use this as an excuse to not eat plenty of vegetables in your plan, but this way if you are low in certain areas such as calcium or iron, you won't have to worry about suffering detrimental health effects because of it.

Greens Supplement

One great alternative and possibly even a better choice than a multi-vitamin is a greens supplement. This one is going to supply you with a good dose of fiber and all the vital nutrients that you'd get from a high intake of fruits and vegetables.

Remember that using this is by no means a substitute for consuming a healthy diet with plenty of fruits and vegetables. By having it as back-up, you can put your mind at ease that you aren't going to be suffering any major deficiencies.

Whey Protein Powder

Another supplement that you may want to look at taking is a good quality whey protein powder. Since protein is the single most important macronutrient for you to be taking as we pointed out earlier, if you're not getting enough you're really going to be suffering.

Since many people do struggle to continuously get in the protein they need, by having a protein powder that you enjoy on hand makes this far easier.

Simply shake with some water and you're all set to go. Protein powder is quick, easy, and often tastes great. With so many different brands and flavours available, you should have no problem finding one that you really enjoy.

In addition to this, protein powder is also especially helpful right before and after your workout since it will get into the muscle tissues quite quickly.

Right at this point you don't want to delay the delivery of amino acids to the muscle cells since it's at this point when they require them the most. Isolate protein powders are designed to rapidly be taken up by the blood stream so by including this specific variety in your pre and post workout meals, you'll definitely boost your recovery ability.

Just do watch that you are using a protein powder however and not a meal replacement powder as these contain far more calories and have a balance of carbs and fats as well. These are fine when you do plan to use them instead of eating a regular meal, but to drink as a source of protein they're going to boost your calorie intake up too high, making staying lean very difficult.

Fish Oil

The next supplement that you'll definitely want to consider adding to your diet is fish oil. Fish oil is extremely helpful on a number of levels from disease prevention to making sure that your body processes and uses carbohydrates correctly.

You'll get these nutrients in any fatty fish sources you consume as well, as we mentioned when discussing the dietary macronutrient fat earlier. If you're someone who doesn't take in a lot of fatty fish on a regular basis, then having this additional supplementation is extremely wise.

Aim for 3-6 grams per day for best benefits, splitting it up into 2-3 doses over the course of the day.

Iron

For some women, supplementing with iron is a very important thing that you should be doing. Iron is a nutrient they often fall short in especially since they're losing some each month with their menstrual cycle and also because since they typically are on much lower total calorie intakes, red meat often gets cut out.

Red meat is by far the most concentrated source of iron in the diet so by restricting this food type, that will definitely cause them to risk falling short.

An iron supplement can quickly make up for this and ensure that energy levels stay at a high throughout the dieting period.

So there you have the main products that you should consider looking at. These will all help to take your overall nutrition up a notch and allow you to see the best benefits from your effort.

Now let's look at a few that you'll want to be very wary of as many people fall into the trap of thinking that they will help them take their results further only to find themselves quickly disappointed.

Fat Burners

The very first and likely one of the most popular supplements by those who are aiming to get leaner are fat burners. Fat burners are composed of a variety of different ingredients and often make very fancy claims about just how much weight they can help you lose.

Keep in mind however that no supplement will ever work magic and many of these claims are just that – claims. Most supplement companies spend more money on their advertising budgets than they do on the scientific research that goes into product development so you can imagine just how effective these really are.

These are often the most problematic supplements as well in terms of distracting you from your overall goals and making you think as though the diet isn't as important as it really is.

Most of those who are using fat burners sometimes assume that the fat burner will take care of the job for them, thus they invest way less effort themselves into the entire process of getting lean.

Don't let yourself fall for this. Most often these fat burners don't help all that much and the little bit they will help out with will just be appetite suppression as well as giving you a boost to your energy levels.

If you do find that you're dragging during your workouts and are quite fatigued, then you may want to consider using them but if you aren't, then there just isn't that need.

Appetite Suppressants

The next type of fat loss product that you may find yourself questioning is an appetite suppressant. These typically claim that they will reduce the feelings of hunger you feel while on a diet, therefore making it easier to stick with the diet plan.

Generally speaking some people do find that these will help, so if hunger is something that you're really battling they may be worth some consideration, but still do keep in mind that you must eat less food in order for them to be effective.

Alone they are not going to make you lose weight – so you still must make sure that you are reducing the number of calories you're taking in overall.

The most common ingredient you'll find in appetite suppressants is hoodia gordonii, however others may be included as well.

Muscle Building products

Finally, the last category of supplements that often receives quite a bit of hype are muscle building products. These include products that claim to help you build muscle and burn fat simultaneously or help to increase your body's stores of muscle building hormones to promote better overall results.

The thing to remember about these is that if you are working towards the goal of fat loss, you aren't going to see large amounts of muscle being built simple because you are not in the calorie surplus that's necessary for you to do so.

While you may find that they help to boost the overall intensity of your workout program, they aren't going to work some kind of magic and help you build massive amounts of muscle while shedding body fat at the same time.

This would just be wishful thinking and starting to believe this will just throw you off course.

If you want to lose fat, focus on fat loss. If you want to build muscle, turn your focus there. Give 100% of your full effort to a single goal and then evaluate how you're progressing along and make some changes accordingly.

So there you have some of the background information that you need to remember when it comes to supplements. Without a doubt there are a few supplements that will help you get closer to reaching your goals but you need to understand which ones they are (and most often they are the least 'fancy' supplements) and then you also must be sure that you're only using them after you have already developed a good diet and workout plan for yourself. When both of those are in place then you have the potential to see good results from adding a supplement to the program.

Remember too that you should always be thoroughly reading the information provided with any supplement you are using and potentially contacting your doctor prior to using them. This is going to go a long way towards ensuring that they are in fact safe for you to use and that you won't experience any harmful interactions with other medications you may be taking.

Most of the basic health related supplements won't pose a threat of this at all so it's not something to be too concerned over, however the performance enhancing ones can sometimes cause issues for those who are very sensitive.

Now that we've covered the supplements section, it's time to move forward and begin discussing the whole other element that will play a role in your fat loss progress – your workout plan.

SECTION 3:
SUPERCHARGING YOUR WORKOUTS FOR FAST AND EFFECTIVE RESULTS

When planning a complete body transformation, there's no question about it – your diet and workout plan are going to work hand in hand. One cannot be as beneficial as possible without the other, so it's vital that you split your time up and pay attention to *both* your workout and diet if you hope to see the results you're after.

Also remember that when your diet is designed properly this will actually support a better overall workout program and you'll see much better results from all your efforts, therefore it's almost like a self-fulfilling cycle.

Put more effort into one area and you will reap benefits in the other because of this. Put less effort and you're asking for some problems.

Now, another important thing that you must keep in mind is that not all exercise is created equally. Some workout programs are far more effective than others, so the key is really discovering which workouts are going to most help you get to your *end result* – as fast as possible.

Remember how we discussed so much in the diet section about forming a meal plan that would help to boost your metabolism so you burn more calories 24/7?

Well, you can do this even more with your workouts. When you're performing the right workouts then you're really going to see that metabolic rate skyrocketing thus weight loss becomes that much easier overall.

We're going to go over all the main things that you should be remembering as you progress through your workouts to ensure that you're doing absolutely everything possible in order to see this taking place.

With a few small adjustments here and there, very often that's all that's needed to really send your results into overdrive.

Let's begin by looking at what the elements are of a proper strength training program.

CHAPTER 17:
WHY WEIGHT LIFTING IS SO IMPORTANT FOR FAT LOSS RESULTS

When most people hear 'weight lifting' they don't automatically associate this with fat loss. Instead, they start thinking about bigger men who utilize weight lifting as a way to pack on more muscle mass and build their body up to a much greater size.

Right now, you really must change your perception of this. While weight lifting is definitely something that you can use to increase the overall size of the body and add more lean muscle mass to your frame in high proportions, that's definitely not all that it will do.

Quite in fact, weight lifting is by far the single most important form of exercise that you could do if you want to see fat loss for a number of reasons.

Let's take a brief look at why weight lifting is so important for fat loss results.

Speeds Metabolism

By far the biggest benefit to weight training is that it will, to a much larger extent than any cardio training, help to boost up your metabolic rate immediately after the session is finished.

While with a cardio workout you may burn 20-30 calories or so after the workout is completed, with weight training, you can literally remain burning calories at an elevated pace for hours once it's completed.

This effect, day after day after day, can then really have quite the influence on the fat loss progress you make because that day to day calorie burn is that much higher.

If you perform three weight lifting workouts a week, this could very well mean your metabolism would stay elevated for the entire weekly time period over and above that of what it normally would be.

Firms and Tones The Body

Second, the next major reason why weight lifting definitely comes in superior to other forms of exercise in terms of making positive improvements to your body is because it's going to really help you firm and tone all the major muscle groups.

While cardio training, if you do it in the form that has you working against resistance (such as uphill walking, biking against resistance, or using the elliptical trainer) can potentially allow you to firm the muscles slightly since they will still be targeted, weight lifting has far more advantages in this area over that of cardio training.

This means that while cardio work can slightly improve the way you look, when you're on a proper resistance training program the results will be that much more noticeable.

Decreases The 'Boredom' Factor

Finally, the last reason why strength training is the much better form of exercise to be performing when aiming for weight loss is because it's also going to significantly help reduce that 'boredom' factor.

Ever been slaving away on the treadmill for forty-five minutes to an hour and become so bored you wished with every ounce of your being you could be somewhere else?

This is incredibly common during cardio sessions because they are, in fact, very, very boring. By nature doing the same movement over and over again is quick to grow old which is why strength training really comes in with the advantage.

With it you'll be constantly moving from one type of exercise to the next therefore will never feel this high degree of boredom.

So as you can see, if you want results, strength training is the way to go. Not only will you improve your body more but you're also going to see remarkable health benefits as well from reduced blood pressure, increased lean muscle mass, lowered risk of diseases such as diabetes, and reduced risk of osteoporosis.

There's no question that this is the type of training that should be forming the foundation of your workout program.

Now let's move forward and take a quick look at what the elements of a good strength training program are so you know precisely what needs to be in place for you to have success.

CHAPTER 18:
THE ELEMENTS OF A PROPER RESISTANCE TRAINING PROGRAM

While there are plenty of ways that you can go about performing an effective strength training routine, there are a few common elements that absolutely must be in place.

If you aren't paying attention to these then you won't be making the gains you could be from your program so it's important to review them so you understand what they are.

When these three elements are in place, that's when your results will increase and you will move closer to the body you're after.

1. Overloading Stimulus

The very first thing that absolutely must be in place for you to see the results you're after is what's called an overloading stimulus. Put quite simply this is some type of stressor on the body that is something you have never seen before or that you can't quite handle comfortably.

It'd be like asking you to learn a new math equation without ever encountering it in the class previously. Since you've never seen it, your brain is going to gain new knowledge, make new connections, and become smarter because of it (assuming, of course, you understand how to do the equation!)

Just like this, with strength training, you're looking to place a task on the body that it has to sit up and react to by either growing stronger, faster, or more powerful.

If you do this consecutively over and over again across time, that's when you're going to see strength gains taking place.

Note that this overloading stimulus can come from a variety of different sources. It doesn't necessarily have to be more and more weight added to the bar because this is quite in fact difficult to do each and every session.

It's unrealistic to expect yourself to make these kind of continual strength gains because doing so would mean we would have some incredibly strong people in this world. Rather, you'll see staggered strength gains where some sessions you do bump up the weight by five to ten pounds and other sessions you've levelled off for a period of weeks even.

When you can't increase the weight to make these strength gains, then you are to look for other ways to increase the overloading stimulus. This can come from places such as increasing the total number of reps you're doing, increasing the number of sets being performed, reducing back on the amount of rest taken in between each set that you do, or adding some more advanced techniques such as supersets, trisets, drop sets, or compound sets, all of which you will learn and utilize when working with an End Result Fitness trainer. Adding these advanced techniques are really what will push your results to the limit so definitely what you should be focusing on once you get that foundation built within the first few months of training.

The important thing to remember is that as you go about your training you should be aiming to slowly change the workout so that something becomes slightly more difficult. If you do that then you'll not only be progressing better but you'll also be preventing a training plateau from occurring as well.

2. Rest

So once this overloading training stimulus has been applied to your workout, then the next thing that must be in place is some rest. If you don't take the time off to let the body recover, you can't really expect results to take place.

One very important thing that many people miss when it comes to succeeding in their gym workouts is the fact that progress actually takes place when you're *outside* of the gym, not inside.

When you're at the gym working hard you're actually slowly breaking down the muscle tissues, making yourself weaker than you were before.

But once those muscle tissues have been broken down and rest is given, that's when you'll grow back stronger than you were before and see the training gains taken place.

If you fail to give the body this rest that it needs however, then what happens is that you just continually go back into the gym after each session, further breaking those tissues down.

Do this often enough and before you know it, you've actually begun to lose muscle tissue rather than build it.

Rest is absolutely essential if you are to see results. Remember too that rest means rest. Some people will think that they can do their hard lifting workout one day and then go do an hour long cardio workout the next, then hit the gym the day following, then go back to doing more cardio, and so on and so forth.

While you can certainly include some cardio training within the weight lifting workouts you're doing, you must be careful to still pay attention to how much overall rest you're getting.

By far the most important rest will be resting that exact muscle group that's being worked, but any stress on the body is still going to tax it and eat into your recovery ability.

Remember that you should never be working a single muscle group two days in a row, but rather allowing for at least 48 hours of rest between the two workouts.

Ideally you should still have at least one full day off a week where you aren't doing anything other than light, leisurely walking.

3. Nutrition

Finally, the last must that needs to be in place is proper nutrition. Nutrition is essentially what will supply the body with the building blocks you need to see that recovery take place.

While rest is definitely enough to jumpstart the process, if you don't provide amino acids for the structure of the muscle tissues as well as glucose for energy for the repair process to take place, your recovery is going to be significantly limited.

Since you will obviously be eating meals throughout the day eventually the body will get the nutrition it needs but you must remember that there's what's referred to as a 'recovery window' immediately after the workout where the body just takes up those nutrients that much more quickly.

Miss this and you're already at a disadvantage. Unfortunately though, as we already discussed in the myths section, many people incorrectly believe that by skipping their nutrition at this point they're actually boosting their overall fat loss progress, which couldn't be further from the truth.

Protein and carbs – in fast digesting sources such as protein powder and simple sugars – are a must for after your hard resistance training workout. If you give your body this, you'll be feeling better faster and will be able to get right back into the gym more quickly to keep at your progress.

So there you have the three main components that make up an effective strength training program. Notice how they all are somewhat integrated together and will work in unison to move you closer to the body you hope to obtain.

If you don't provide the overloading stimulus, there's no real need to have that rest period since the recovery process isn't nearly as extreme (muscle tissue won't be broken down). Likewise, if you don't provide the rest for recovery, chances are you won't be able to apply that overloading stimulus either as the body simply won't be able to keep up to the previous demands being placed on it and move forward to more advanced, higher level stressors.

Finally, if nutrition isn't applied, then you won't have the energy to workout in the gym either, so once again, the entire cycle moves out of balance.

When all three are effectively working together though, that's when you start seeing the amazing results you've been looking for.

Now we're going to move forward and talk about a few different methods of performing your resistance training, outlining which one tends to be the most effective.

CHAPTER 19:
METHODS OF RESISTANCE TRAINING

When it comes to including resistance training in your workout program, there is a wide array of opportunities to perform exercises that will stimulate the body in this manner.

With many advancements in the fitness field, new equipment is coming out regularly that will challenge the muscles and add more interest to your workout program.

In looking through all these different pieces of equipment however, it's still very essential that you are evaluating them for their actual benefits to the body.

Just like various types of exercise will offer different levels of effectiveness, various types of equipment will also play a role in how you progress along.

Without question some forms of equipment are far superior to others so by using those more often you can jumpstart the results you see.

Let's quickly go over what you do want in a workout program.

Unstable Environment

The very first thing that you'll want to be sure is in place is that you're creating an unstable environment for yourself. What this essentially means is that as you go about any of your strength based exercises, your body is slightly off balance.

Because of this fact, every single muscle fiber not only in the target muscles you're aiming to work but also throughout the entire core of the body must contract rapidly to maintain your balance.

As this occurs, you're not only going to burn more calories per minute but you're also going to get that much stronger. This dynamic type of motion that has you constantly moving around and correcting yourself is also an ideal way to work on your agility and coordination, so anyone interested in improving those two aspects of their fitness level will really benefit as well.

Any form of exercise performed on a stability ball, a bosu ball, incorporating in the use of a medicine ball, or done on the FreeMotion line of equipment will accomplish the unstable environment objective perfectly.

Self-Directed Action Patterns

On the other hand, what you don't want is to get into a piece of equipment that essentially locks you into place while you perform the movement, giving you little to no room for self-adjustment.

This not only puts many muscles in the body 'to sleep' as they don't need to be contracting to maintain your position but it can also set you up for an injury as well.

Due to the fact that these machines will already have your movement pattern set, if they don't quite fit your body properly, this could mean it not only feels uncomfortable for you to move through but that you stress the body in a way you shouldn't.

Injuries are extremely common when relying just on machines to do the workout so this is something that you really want to do your best to avoid.

Free weights are always going to be superior to machines in this regard so they are what you should be focusing your workout around.

Maximum Muscle Recruitment

The third must have for a proper strength training program as far as equipment selection goes and the type of workout you're performing is one where you're aiming to recruit a maximum number of muscle fibers per exercise.

This is going to be done very efficiently whenever you're performing compound lifts, which is in opposition to isolation movements.

Free weights naturally tend to be more compound in nature even if you are performing an exercise such as bicep curls because even still you will be using your ab muscles there to maintain your upright position.

If you were sitting in a machine performing the same exercise there's absolutely no activation necessary throughout the core therefore these muscles go dormant.

Don't think you necessarily need to always turn to weights to accomplish compound exercises either. There are plenty of bodyweight exercises that can be performed as you go about your program that will likewise work a number of muscle fibers at once and really up your strength level and calorie burn.

You'll want to take note that this is also what makes the Jacobs Ladder, which you'll definitely use when working with a trainer at End Result Fitness so effective. It's going to target all the largest muscles in the body such as the back, delts, quads, hamstrings, and glutes, while still working the arms, abs, and calves all at the same time.

The result of this is that our users see better results than any other form of cardio training – even a high intensity run. This means you'll have to spend far less time doing your cardio training to get the results that you're after.

Variety

Finally, the last thing that's important to have within the context of your resistance training program is variety. The body is going to react best when the stressor is constantly changing so it's vital that you never let yourself get too complacent with your workout routine.

When you're using exercise equipment such as dumbbells, stability balls, adjustable benches, medicine balls, and the FreeMotion dual cable cross, you'll have a never-ending supply of exercises that can be performed.

This makes it much more enjoyable to complete your daily sessions and will also help to prevent any muscular imbalances due to you neglecting any given muscle on the body.

When working with a trainer at End Result Fitness the exercises will constantly be changing so you will never have to worry that you aren't going to stress the muscles in a variety of different ways.

So there you have the main factors that must be taken into consideration when selecting your method of resistance training.

While you could rely on just a single one of these methods – free weights, using just a stability ball or medicine ball, or strictly sticking with the FreeMotion equipment, you'll see the absolute best results when you combine them all together.

Also note that this isn't to say you can't get results using other types of equipment – if you're dead set on machines and it's the only thing that makes you feel comfortable in the gym, so be it.

It's just that if you want to see the most optimal results possible, then these are the variations that are strongly recommended. It all does come down to your comfort factor and goal set so these issues will all have to be taken into consideration.

Now that you can clearly see which type of resistance training is the most beneficial for results, let's spend some time discussing some of the important parameters that you should keep in mind when designing an effective workout program.

CHAPTER 20:
SETTING THE PARAMETERS OF YOUR RESISTANCE TRAINING PROGRAM

After you have your equipment selection in place, the next step in designing a workout program is to look at the various elements that determine how you go about doing this workout itself.

When working with a trainer at End Result Fitness, this will be carefully calculated based on your needs, goals, current fitness level, and the general shape and structure of your body.

All of these factors will go into determining the optimal training selection for your body that will help you ensure top-level results.

Many people are quick to adopt the 'standard' set of training parameters and then don't see the results they could because of this. It's one other big reason why working with a trainer really does prove to be superior.

This also isn't to mention the fact that these parameters should ideally be constantly changing as you go about your program and progress through, so that's another drawback that many people face if they're just selecting a workout out of some magazine or other read-made source.

Complete customization is what you want in order to reach your body composition goals.

But, let's dig deeper into these parameters so you can understand what they're all about and how they are going to impact you.

Reps and Sets

The very first thing that you must decide upon is how many reps and sets you're going to perform for each exercise. For those of you who aren't quite up on the 'fitness lingo', reps refers to how many times you're going to lift a weight up and move it back down to the starting position while sets refers to how many sequences of these reps you perform.

Usually there is a somewhat inverse relationship between how many sets are performed and how many reps are executed as this is what will help ensure that the total volume (which is reps X sets X weight lifted) stays in an ideal zone.

If you're doing very high reps and also doing very high sets, chances are you're going to begin overtaxing the body and will not recover optimally.

Now, at End Result Fitness the focused rep range will vary slightly depending on the particular phase of the program you're in and what your specific goal is at the time, but you will be mostly focused on lifting somewhere between eight and twelve reps, which will stimulate not only that metabolic increase that we've referred to before but will also help to add more muscle definition and get you looking leaner. I would make the rep range much broader.

In addition to this, at some points in the program you may be working with your trainer who takes you up to a rep range of 25 reps per exercise and this will also be another great way to stimulate the muscle tissue from a different perspective.

Remember, the best results will come from a wide variety of training methods so your trainer will be sure to switch it up frequently so you can get to your *end result*.

If you are very focused on generating strength, then we will move this rep range slightly lower so you can lift more weight total however this will still be combined with some sets performed in the slightly higher rep range.

Time and time again we've seen our clients progress at this rep range the best and the scientific research is there to prove it, so it's clearly the right way to go.

When sets get factored in, you'll be performing slightly more sets when doing your compound exercises than any isolation movements that may be added into the program for the fact that these not only work more muscle fibers total but also because they are simply going to be more effective overall.

You always want to spend the greater proportion of time during your workout focused on what will get you the fastest and most predominant results, which is precisely what we do at End Result Fitness.

You may find that some other trainers will use a number of isolations within their workouts but all this does is reduce back on the progress that's made. Sure, you may have slightly more variety in the workout program but we strongly believe that results are the end goal here.

With our workouts you'll get enough variety to keep it interesting while making sure that every single second in your workout program is geared towards delivering progress. Why spend two weeks working on achieving something that you could have done in a single week?

That is our philosophy. Always use the *most effective* training methods to get the *fastest results possible.*

Rest Periods

Moving on, another element of the workout program that needs to get assessed is the amount of rest you're taking between each set that you perform.

Here again, when working with a trainer at End Result Fitness you'll find this does vary depending on what you're doing. Different exercises and training methods will place far different stress levels on the body so when working with your personal trainer they will automatically adjust the rest range to what's required for your body to recover.

As you begin to use some of the advanced lifting techniques that we've mentioned earlier including things like supersets or drop sets, your rest periods will vary again since this throws a whole other form of stimulus on the body.

The one thing that's for certain though is that rest can have a significant influence on your ability to lift a proper amount of weight, so it's not something that you can afford to overlook. If you aren't using proper rest periods, not only will you not get the fat burning hormonal release from your workouts that you could be seeing but you will also fatigue out much quicker and may not even be able to complete the workout itself.

Far too many people don't account for rest and just go by what 'feels best' and this could be one of the biggest mistakes that's holding you back from progress.

Your trainer will work with you to figure out whether you require 30 seconds, 60 seconds, or 2 minutes between your sets, or whether you are going to move directly from exercise to exercise instead.

It's also important to keep in mind that at times you may use an active recovery technique where you stimulate smaller muscle groups while larger ones are resting.

These muscle groups don't require as much oxygen in order to recover like the larger muscle groups do when you perform compound exercises so your program will be structured to identify with that fact.

Workout Program Design

Third, the next element to consider is the overall workout program design and set-up. This refers to how you go about structuring the days you work each muscle group in the body.

For instance, the main types of workout programs you'll come across are full body workouts, upper/lower split workouts, and body part split workouts.

When doing a full body workout you're going to be stimulating each and every muscle in the body with every workout that you do, which then means you can work each area two to three times a week (since at least one day off must be taken between sessions).

If you're doing an upper/lower split design however, then you'll be hitting the upper body twice per week and only performing movements for this region of the body on those days and then coupling this with two lower body workouts as well.

The advantage here is that you can perform slightly more exercises for each muscle group since you are splitting the body up in half but the drawback is that the most you'll hit each muscle is twice per week.

Finally, body part splits are where you just work a single muscle group each day you're in the gym, usually only hitting it once per week.

At End Result Fitness, we strongly believe in the full body approach since it's going to be the best in terms of boosting your BMR (allowing you to burn more calories 24/7) and will help to deliver the utmost fastest results.

This full body approach is also going to help provide a greater BMR increase to the body since you're stimulating all the main large muscle groups at once and forcing your body to work to such a high intensity.

For instance, when you're doing your workout session, if you include leg exercises into the mix, you'll burn up to ten times more calories than when doing arm exercise thus indicating just how essential large muscle group training is for fat loss.

By doing the full body workout we are sure to hit your legs with each and every workout therefore really spiking your calorie burn and moving you that much closer to your *end result*.

If you are at a slightly more advanced level in your training however then the trainer you work with may put you on a more intricate type of set-up where you are doing just upper or lower body in the gym with End Result Fitness on some days and then doing a full body workout at home yourself on other days.

This will all be determined in session after your goals have been outlined and progress has been assessed.

Very rarely are body part split workouts utilized as targeting only a single muscle group on the body. This is not going to have you burning up many calories at all and will make things very difficult from a frequency standpoint. Once you try and factor in your cardio training into this type of design, it gets very tricky from a scheduling point of view.

Weight Lifted

Finally, the last aspect of your workout program that must get looked at is how much weight you'll be lifting.

One thing that we must stress at this point is that you should not be afraid to lift a heavier weight.

This is one of the biggest mistakes that many people make, especially women who are under the belief that they're going to get big and bulky.

We've already mentioned this earlier but it's worth stating again – women simply do not have the hormonal environment to build up large amounts of muscle mass quickly so you can put that fear right out of your mind.

Lifting a weight that fully challenges you within the rep range recommended by your trainer is what will cause the metabolism to skyrocket and allow you to get that muscle tone.

Think of it this way – if you aren't lifting a weight that challenges the muscles, why should they change?

They won't. It's that process of the overloading stimulus again.

Whether your trainer has you working in the 8 rep range or going up into the high intensity 25 rep range, you'll still be lifting a weight that really challenges the body so you provide that degree of stimulation.

Keep in mind with this point that in most cases the amount of weight you're actually lifting has a direct relationship to the size of the muscle being worked.

For example, you'll lift far more weight doing a leg exercise than you would a bicep exercise partly due to the sheer number of muscle fibers at work. The more muscle fibers you have powering you through the exercise, the more weight you're able to push.

If you go and try and hoist a 30 pound weight however, then all of a sudden it's unable to handle this job and will react because of it.

You never want to be lifting so heavy that you sacrifice good form, but when you have your first session with your trainer they will go over with you exactly how much weight your body can handle given the exercise and rep range protocol you'll be using.

Guessing and testing in terms of weight lifted can lead to less than optimal progress so this is yet another element where having someone there in person to guide you is beneficial.

When you do, you'll be guaranteed to see results.

So there you have the main basic components of designing a workout program. As you can see it's more than just selecting a few exercises and picking up the weights.

There are numerous factors that must get accounted for that will ensure that you feel your best throughout the workout, recover properly, and start making progress immediately.

If you miss out on any of these elements in your program, you're going to instantly see the disappointing results because of it.

Now let's briefly go over how to go about choosing the best workout for your own situation.

CHAPTER 21:
CHOOSING THE BEST WORKOUT DESIGN FOR YOU

As we've now discussed all the main components of a workout that you need to be keeping in mind, you may be finding yourself feeling a little overwhelmed by all the information and trying to figure out which is the right way to go for you.

This is the single most important reason why it's highly beneficial to have a personal trainer to walk you through this – guidance and reassurance.

When you're with a personal trainer, you can feel confident that you're making the right selection and are moving directly closer to your goals.

When you don't have that assistance, you may find that you're often questioning exactly what it is that you're doing. Fortunately, that's why we're here to help.

Let's have a quick look at some of the main issues that you'll be considering when working with your trainer in choosing which workout program is going to be most ideal for you.

Time Commitment

The very first thing that must get assessed is what your time commitment is like. If you're unable to get into the gym four days a week, putting you on a four day a week program is obviously not going to be a smart move.

The great news is that the trainers at End Result Fitness are able to customize your workout plan to meet your time demands. If you can only hit the gym twice per week, that's fine. We'll work with that.

You must find a way to accommodate your workouts to how much time availability you have present because if you don't, you're going to be facing an uphill battle from the start.

If you have more time available to exercise, then you can spend a little more time each session focused on the various muscle groups.

Whatever situation you happen to be in, this will still not influence whether or not you are able to get results. All it does is change the structure of your program set-up.

Many people who are working on their own however, would have significant issues trying to fit a proper workout into just two sessions, which again is why having the trainer there serves to overcome this difficulty.

Remember, time is the #1 asset that you have in life and you definitely do not want to waste time doing a workout that isn't bringing you the results you want.

You work hard in the gym and deserve to be rewarded so make sure that you are taking the necessary steps such as contacting a trainer at End Result Fitness to make whatever time commitment you can put forth 100% productive.

Skill Level

Second, you must also take a good look at your skill level. Someone who's brand new to fitness and just starting out will be performing many different exercises than someone who has been at it for two to three years already.

Those who are more advanced with their training will need to challenge their body in many different ways if they are going to continue to progress as they should.

Unless you're taking this factor into account and looking at what will be necessary in order for you to reach your goals, the chances are high that you're going to fall short.

Putting someone who is more skilled on a basic program will simply waste their time and lead to frustration and lack of progress.

The trainers at End Result Fitness will look extensively at what your current abilities are and ensure that your program is going to match this.

Exercise Preference

It's also going to be necessary to keep your overall exercise preference in mind. While there will always be some restrictions with this as you simply must be performing certain exercises if you do hope to accomplish your goal, you definitely can tailor a program towards exercises you naturally enjoy.

Cardio proves to be a good illustration of this. Let's say that you, with your whole heart, hate running.

Would it be a good idea to put yourself on a 4-day running program to try and lose weight?

Obviously not. Even if you did manage to stick with it for a few weeks, chances are those few weeks are going to be some of the most frustrating ones in your life.

Thankfully much of the exercises that are incorporated into your workout program with End Result Fitness are more interesting than the average cardio session so this shouldn't be a problem, but still, your preferences are always taken into account.

We know that if you enjoy your workouts, your chances of sticking with it are that much higher, therefore your results will be that much better. This is accounted for greatly in the overall program design.

Goal Set

Finally, the last element that gets factored into determining the optimal workout for you is your goal set. Two people who have very similar goals – say goals of fat loss, may need to approach this from different angles in order to see success.

This will come down largely to certain aspects of your lifestyle and what motivates you to complete a workout and diet program. By talking with your trainer at End Result Fitness, you can discuss the best approach for you to take in order to get to your *end result*.

Customization again here is the key.

So there you have the main things to remember when selecting a workout program that's right for you. When all of these elements are considered, that's when you'll be able to choose between a few of the different workouts you may come across.

It is best to get the opinion of a professional trainer whenever you can since they will have that background knowledge you need coupled with the many years of experience working with a variety of different clients.

Even if you're just doing one or two workouts per week with an End Result Fitness trainer and then plan to do a few workouts on your own time, this will still provide a very nice combination to move you forward with your goals.

Now let's move on and talk a little bit about training differences between males and females.

CHAPTER 22:
TRAINING DIFFERENCES FOR MALES VERSUS FEMALES

One question that many of the clients who come to me often wonder about is whether there is any training differences between males versus females.

Many people firmly believe that since men are much more muscular, they need to be training in a very different manner than a woman does.

Likewise, since women tend to be more petite without that very muscular stature, they feel that again, the training style must vary to prevent the development of too much muscle mass.

The very first thing to remember here is that females will never build up great proportions of muscle tissue unless they work at it for years and years as we've already touched upon and unless they are eating very high volumes of food.

So right now put that thought to rest.

The second thing to think about is the fact that regardless of whether you're male or female, a very similar process of building muscle mass is going to occur. You need to apply some type of overloading stimulus – stress those muscle tissues maximally, allow the body to reset and recover, and also get in proper nutrition.

Those three key elements right there are what will get you to the finish line – YOUR *END RESULT*. This is what we specialize in at End Result Fitness.

Since the basic process is the same for both men and women then there aren't a lot of major differences between the training styles. Both should be lifting a weight that's going to challenge the body (males will typically on average lift more than females will), both should be making sure to design their program using the methods that we've outlined earlier, and both should be being mindful of good rest and nutrition.

Do that and you're going to see progress. That's not to say that there aren't any differences whatsoever in the training requirements for males or females though – there are and we're going to take a look at them right now.

Volume

The very first difference that I find with my male and female clients is the amount of volume that they are able to handle. In 90% of the cases (the other 10% being issues of higher level female athletes compared to males who have never worked out in their lives) men will be able to handle more total volume each workout than women.

Partly this is due to their much greater testosterone levels. Since this hormone is largely involved in the muscle building process it also plays a significant role in how much you can handle per workout sessions.

Those males who have very high testosterone levels may find that they can do upwards of 30 sets or more each workout while females who have very low levels of testosterone (which is normal) may only be able to do 15-20.

This then makes a difference in the overall structure and set-up of the workout program and should be adjusted accordingly.

When you work with us at End Result Fitness, we'll be carefully assessing exactly how much volume is necessary for you to see the best possible results from your program without pushing you to become over trained.

This careful balance is absolutely vital and is a huge reason why I do really recommend working with a trainer. If you don't understand how much volume your body can handle and do start to do too much, you'll actually move backwards rather than forwards.

But on the flip side, if you're not doing enough volume in your training, that's also going to work against you as well as you won't be applying enough of that necessary stimulus needed for overall muscle improvements.

It's a very fine line that you have to be walking on and at End Result Fitness we will help you find it perfectly.

Recovery and Recuperation

Second, the next training difference between males and females is going to be your level of recovery. Again, this goes back to testosterone (you can see a trend forming here!). Since men have more testosterone in their bodies, they're usually able to recover faster between workout sessions, therefore can not only tolerate a higher amount of volume but are also able to tolerate more frequent workout sessions.

If you're a female and are finding yourself dragging from workout to workout, this is a sign that full recovery is not taking place. It's also one reason why you're going to find when you work with us you're focusing on only those exercises that really work many muscle groups in the body.

By using these, you'll cut down on how much time you must spend exercising but still see very good results – better results in fact than if you would have done more.

Basically, you're getting *more for less*. More results for less total work. We've develop a precise strategy for our workouts to make this happen.

Males are also more likely to adopt a type of training set-up where a few more exercises are performed for specific muscle groups that they really want to focus on growing larger but they can handle that added volume.

If you're a male who wants to see improvements in your chest, biceps, or back so you can get that 'V' tapered look that makes you look masculine and powerful, when you come to workout with us we'll be setting you up on a specific program that is going to really target those areas.

That's not to say you won't work the rest of your body – you will be but we'll also make sure that your side goal for that specific part is met.

So there's the second difference between men and women. Recovery is such an important element in the equation for success so it's something you really must understand carefully when going about your workout program.

Exercise Preference

Moving on, another key difference that's often noticed with men and women is their overall exercise preference. I've worked with numerous female clients who very strongly gravitate to the cardio-based forms of training.

Usually, this is because that's what they've always done up until this point – that's what they *know*. Hence, they figure that's their way to their *end result*.

Sadly though, it isn't and usually it takes a good convincing from myself or one of the other professional trainers at End Result Fitness to show them otherwise.

Males on the other hand naturally tend to gravitate to more strength based movements because for them, building strength and adding muscle has always been the focus.

I'll definitely see males who have the goal to lose body fat but still, they are always interested in their weight lifting or resistance training workouts.

Most females will shy away at first until we ease them into it and they begin to see how great of results they can get when they add that strength training element into their program plan.

Exercise Selection

Finally, the last big difference that comes about with male versus female training is the exercise selection that's used.

It never fails that when my female clients come to me they want to either firm their abs, tone their underarms, or get rid of their 'saddlebags' that they've noticed have started to develop over the years.

Due to the fact that men and women tend to naturally store body fat in different regions of the body, this is going to effect the type of results they are looking for.

A man may want to slim down his waistline while the woman is more concerned with her hips.

Most males also tend to have relatively leaner upper bodies (assuming they are at a reasonable body fat level) while for females this is a big problem area. Those under arms especially will be a place where 70% of women store much of their body fat so really looking into exercises that will target this region will be vital.

Since we know each person has a different *end result* they are going for, we will completely customize the program to accomplish your particular goals.

Men and women will require a few slightly different exercises so that you can zero in and target those particular trouble zones.

The focus should still largely be on lifting with compound exercises, using metabolic training to help you burn more calories all day long, as well as applying all the other principles we discussed above to get you to your *end result*. The only difference is that now you're really making sure that the exercises you do perform will specifically work that area as well.

That sums up the main training differences between males and females. For the most part, both genders can do very similar program designs and will both respond in a highly favourable manner to the workouts we put you on.

The key is customizing your program to your own individual preferences and desires while staying within the realm of effective training. Since that's what we specialize in at End Result Fitness, you can rest assured that your progress will be in good hands.

Now we're going to move on and look at some advanced workout techniques that you can use to boost your level of progress and take things to the next level.

You will be integrating many of these into your program when you train with us at End Result Fitness. You are going to be placing a much higher level of stress on the body and it's going to be extremely important that you're doing this correctly.

Some misjudgement in going about these techniques or a failure to follow proper form could very quickly lead to injury as well as numerous other problems so it's something that absolutely must be held in check.

CHAPTER 23:
ADVANCED WORKOUT TECHNIQUES TO BOOST PROGRESS

Once you've been at your workouts for a while and feel like you're ready to bump up the intensity and really take a step in the right direction of achieving success, following advanced workout techniques will stimulate those muscles and get you looking your best.

It's important not to dive into these until you have a good fitness base built as that's what will prepare you for what's to come.

Remember, progression – at a rate that's constant but realistic for you is what will get you your *end result*.

If you try and push yourself too hard too soon, all that will wind up happening is you'll dislike exercise and may even get injured. Take it day by day moving further and further closer to your goal and when you're ready for the advanced workout techniques we're about to describe, your body will tell you.

Let's take a look at the techniques to consider.

Supersets

The first technique for adding that extra intensity into your workout program are supersets. Supersets are great to shorten up your workout, get your heart rate up, help you burn calories faster than ever, and improve how many calories you burn after the workout is completed as well.

For most people who are currently advancing from the more basic beginners workout program into something more advanced, this is one of the best ways to start. Most people will quickly pick on how to do these and can add one, two, or three different supersets into their workout without too much trouble.

When looking at the actual superset itself, what you'll be doing is pairing two exercises back to back taking no rest in between. Then once that second set is completed, then comes your rest period before proceeding to do it one more time.

Usually you'll take two exercises that work opposing muscle groups and put them together (such as a chest press and bent over row for instance), however sometimes you may also pair two exercises for the same body part together.

Do note that this latter technique is much more intense since that particular muscle is really working for an extended period of time so if that's your strategy, you must be ready for it. You won't be able to do as many of these sets in your workout program without burning out so start slowly.

Drop Sets

The next way of boosting the intensity in your workout program is to add in some drop sets. What a drop set will be is where you perform one exercise at your usual weight for the desired number of sets(say your dumbbell chest press for 15 reps at 20 pounds) and then immediately drop the weight down a notch after that set is complete and move on to a second set at 15 or 10 pounds. Do one complete set of 8 at that weight and then drop the weight one more time and try and do a third set.

This technique is really great for inducing a higher state of overall muscle fatigue in the tissue and is going to be effective to help you bust through a training plateau. When training for maximum fat loss you want to be sure that you keep challenging the muscle tissues on an ongoing basis because this is what will keep the metabolism higher and allow you to continue to burn fat.

Plus, if you then also build up a small amount of lean muscle tissue in the process, this will mean that you will burn more calories 24 hours a day without having to do any extra exercise. It's really a powerful tool in the fat loss formula.

After you do a few weeks of this type of training, you'll likely find that when you go to do a straight set at a higher weight (say a set of 15 at 25 pounds), now it's possible.

Again with drop sets remember that they are going to bump up the volume of your workout program significantly so that must be factored into it as well so that you don't begin to overtrain yourself.

Tri-Sets

Tri-sets are the third way of boosting the intensity and are essentially the superset's more intense cousin.

Now rather than taking two exercises and pairing them back to back, you're taking *three exercises* and doing them one right after another.

This is verging on more of a circuit training fashion with the workout – which is fine. The point is that it will increase the metabolic rate, improve your body's ability to withstand fatigue, and get you great results.

Just don't expect to hit any strength records on that last exercise when using trisets because you're definitely going to notice fatigue is kicking in.

You could pair three exercises for the same muscle group in this tri-set but the more common approach is to either hit three different muscle groups throughout it. Often you'll do a lower body exercise and then immediately after that move into two upper body exercises after that, or you may do a compound exercise and follow that with two more isolated exercises that work muscle groups that were targeted within that compound lift.

However you choose to set it up, you can be sure that this will definitely challenge your muscles to quite a large extent.

Pre-Fatigue

Finally our last way to challenge your muscles further is going to be by adding an element of pre-fatigue to the mix. With this type of technique the objective is to enhance the results from a compound movement by tiring out one of the helper muscles involved in that movement, thus forcing the main muscle to be worked that much harder.

So for instance, using dumbbell chest press as an example once again, if you're really looking for some serious chest gains, you may consider performing some tricep extensions first since the triceps are going to be helping you execute the bench press, making sure they are fatigued and then move directly to your chest press exercise.

Now when you move over and do that you'll notice that the triceps are no longer helping like they used to thus more stress is placed on that chest muscle, ramping up the amount of stimulus it receives – and accomplishing your primary objective.

When doing pre-fatigue sets though you do want to make sure you have your spotter around for safety. If you're tired and lifting a heavy weight on compound movements and fail to get the weight back up, the risk of injury is going to be that much weaker.

Don't be surprised if you do actually go down in weight when moving to that compound lift compared to what you'd lift if you were doing a straight set as you essentially have a lower level of muscular force behind you.

So there you have some of the key components to upping the intensity of your workout and moving you closer to achieving your desired *end result*.

Below I'm going to show you a sample workout program that essentially takes a basic beginner level program and moves it into a more intermediate level and then advanced workout program. Obviously this would be completely customized for you when you work with a trainer at End Result Fitness but this should give you a bit of an idea how the overall set-up works.

Beginner Full Body Workout

Superset: Squats with Dumbbell Chest Press – 2 sets of 12-15
Superset: Bent Over Dumbbell Rows with Lunges– 2 sets of 12-15
Superset: Step-ups with Shoulder Press – 2 sets of 12-15
Crunches On An Exercise Ball – 2 sets of 12-15

Intermediate Full Body Workout

Superset: Squats with Deadlifts – 3 sets of 12-15
Superset: Dumbbell Chest Press with Bent Over Row – 3 sets of 12-15
Superset: Pull-Ups with Lateral Raise -3 sets of 12-15
Triset: Lunges, Bicep Curls, Tricep Extensions - 3 sets of 12-15
Superset: Crunches on an Exercise Ball with Lying Leg Raises – 3 sets of 12-15

Advanced Full Body Workout

Pre-Fatigue Superset: Tricep Extensions with Bench Press – 3 sets of 12-15
Pre-Fatigue Superset: Lunges with Squats – 3 sets of 12-15
Superset: Shoulder Press with Lateral Raise – 3 sets of 12-15
Pre-Fatigue Superset: Bicep Curls with Pull-Ups – 3 sets of 12-15
Superset: Bent Over Rows with Reverse Fly's – 3 sets of 12-15
Triset: Crunches on an Exercise Ball, Lying Leg Raise, Plank – 3 sets of 12-15

When it comes to the point that you're feeling like you could be doing more with your workout program and seeing better results, it's always a good idea to discuss your thoughts with your trainer at End Result Fitness.

Then we will work with you to come up with a solution to move forward towards your goals and make sure you see the *end result* you're after.

This is one of the major benefits of working with a trainer – constant progression. We'll be carefully watching for signs that you're in need of a challenge as you do your workouts and you'll advance naturally as we alter your program as you go.

Remember when you work with one of our trainers, no two workouts will ever be exactly alike so all of the concepts I just discussed will be integrated in for you.

Now that we're finished our progress discussion, let's talk about another issue that must be addressed – the plateau.

If you're currently not satisfied with the rate you're progressing with your workouts that you're currently doing alone at the moment, it helps to know what you can do to bust past this plateau and start moving ahead once again.

CHAPTER 24:
HOW TO BEAT A TRAINING PLATEAU

One of the single most frustrating things that anyone can experience with regards to their workout program is the training plateau. You're moving ahead great – seeing the scale going down, noticing positive changes in how your body looks, and feeling better than ever, when all of a sudden it just stops.

Confused, uncertain, and more than likely upset, this leaves you wondering what you're doing wrong.

Training plateaus are by far one of the most common reasons that our clients approach us at End Result Fitness. They've usually been doing some form of workout program on their own for a brief period of time but lately just have not been getting the results they were after.

It's at this point that they realize, they need help.

Fortunately, this is what we're all about – getting you to your *end result*. Unless you understand the key fundamentals of making sure the muscle tissues are overloaded in the right way, a plateau is virtually inevitable. It will happen at one point or another and you will grow frustrated.

When you're with a trainer however, the variability and constant progress is built right into the program hence you avoid it altogether.

Prevention is always the best medicine and our programs are designed with this in mind.

To illustrate this concept, we may have you doing 3 sets of 25 reps for one exercise one week and then the next week, you'd move over to a 4 sets of 12 rep scheme. This entirely changes the stressor on the muscles and will promote constant muscle development.

You must realize that your body encompasses multiple areas of fitness and to only challenge it across one level would be a huge mistake. Rather, you should be taking pure strength, muscular endurance, muscular flexibility, and aerobic conditioning in mind, integrating all of these elements into a single workout program that will get you a higher level of results.

When you miss out on some element of these components, that's when you're going to see gaps occurring in your progress and those plateau's setting in.

Once again, this is where End Result Fitness trainers will help you overcome this. We'll target every single aspect of your fitness level within our workouts so you never have to worry about this issue.

All you have to worry about is putting in the hard effort and then enjoying the results that are going to come.

Remember that there are numerous ways to push through a plateau including changing the exercises around, altering the reps and sets to be performed, changing the entire workout split (so you're working out more frequently or less frequently depending on the design of the overall workout program) or throwing some new equipment into the mix.

Our trainers are accustomed to using a variety of different methods with their clients so you will touch upon all aspects throughout your time working out with us.

Let's now move on and discuss another critical issue that you must be aware about if you're going to have success with our workouts – overtraining.

CHAPTER 25:
PREVENTING OVERTRAINING SYNDROME

If there's one thing that will really set you back in your progress, becoming overtrained is it.

Overtraining is a very real issue and many people mistakenly think that it's only going to happen to high level athletes or fitness competitors.

Not so.

Anyone – even the most basic beginner can experience overtraining if they aren't careful with how they're designing their workout program and this issue can potentially take you right out of your workouts altogether.

The main reason overtraining occurs in the body is simple: you're presenting your body with an overloading stress that it's simply unable to keep up to.

In short, it can't handle the recovery. You are doing too much work for what your body is able to tolerate and it's not having that chance to repair itself and grow back stronger.

Hence, as you move through your workout thinking you're doing the right thing by continuing on and pushing hard, you're actually just further breaking the body down and making it weaker and weaker.

Over time, the body may become so weak that it actually starts to lose lean muscle mass. When that happens, that's when you're in for some real trouble.

Learning to recognize some of the symptoms of overtraining is a good place to start so you can work to combat this problem. Prevention is definitely going to be your best strategy here (which we'll get to in a second) so by learning to spot when the signs are showing themselves that you may be on the verge of overtraining, you can reverse the situation and get yourself back on track again.

Let's take a look at the most important signals to watch out for.

High Levels Of Fatigue

The very first marker to be aware of when it comes to overtraining is a high level of fatigue. Usually this is the one that will set most people off that something may be up and it's noticeable fairly soon once the condition begins to develop.

If you're finding that you're going into your workouts each day and are feeling more tired with each successive session, something needs to be changed.

The first thing to do in this instance is to evaluate your sleep and your diet. If it has only occurred once or twice then it could be a simple fix of going to bed an hour earlier or making sure that you get in a few more carbs before your workout.

It's when the fatigue has persisted for at least a week or longer though that you really want to sit up and take notice. In this case it's likely not just a situation factor that's causing the problem but is something larger than that.

Note that this fatigue does not need to be just limited to your workout session either. In fact, in some cases it's the opposite that happens. You get into the gym and the endorphins get running through your system and suddenly you do have enough energy to get through the workout.

But then after the workout is completed, it's then that you feel like all you can do is lay on the couch and not move. You're wiped right out.

If this describes you, that's a very good indication that you may just be pushing yourself a little too hard in the gym.

It's good to be tired after a hard workout but you shouldn't be so tired that you're rendered practically useless.

Poor Performance

The second thing to look at is what your performance level is like. This obviously goes hand in hand with the fatigue issue because when you're highly fatigued and tired, that will have a direct impact on the performance you put forth.

If you notice that your strength levels are really decreasing and you're muscular endurance has also gone downhill (you can't complete as many sets or reps as you normally would) that can be a good sign that overtraining could be at play.

There are definitely going to be those days where you are just not into your workout and can't really put the amount of effort that you normally would Once again we're looking for longer term trends here, not just that day to day fatigue that can happen based on what else you have going on in your life. If you're performance is on a steady decline rather than a steady incline, something's up.

Increased Irritability

Moving away from your actual workout sessions, the next issue that you may run into is a greatly increased amount of irritability. Those who are verging on becoming overtrained will show both physiological as well as psychological changes and will often become really quite irritable.

Those who are usually around them on a regular basis may make comments that they aren't their typical selves and are easily agitated by little everyday occurrences.

Mood changes are definitely normal when overtraining sets in so that's something that you clearly do need to be aware of.

Weight Gain or Loss

Another issue that may come about when you're moving into an overtrained state is weight gain or weight loss. Usually this is accompanied by an appetite change thus it directly effects your overall body weight.

In most situations it's actually an appetite loss that occurs so that's what to really look out for but it can work the other way in some instances.

The main thing you're looking for is a change from the norm. If you are training very intensity and recently boosted up the training, it is normal to experience a higher level of hunger because of this. If you haven't changed your training all that much but have notice a significant incline in appetite, that's your signal to look further into the situation.

Difficulty Sleeping

If you start to find that you're tossing and turning in bed on a regular basis and just can't seem to make it through a good night's sleep, this too can indicate that overtraining could be coming into play.

When the body is so highly stressed from an overload of both exercise as well as other factors that could be creeping up in your lifestyle, you're going to notice that you just aren't getting the quality of rest that you were hoping for.

Since rest is the primary time when the body is going to be under that high repair process, if you aren't getting rest, you're in trouble.

You should always be sleeping at least seven hours each night (eight hours is better) and when you aren't getting this in, trouble is going to creep up.

Being Uninterested In Everyday Activities

One symptom that often will present itself once overtraining is already taking place (it won't be as present beforehand when you're just becoming overtrained) is the feeling of being uninterested in activities that you typically would have enjoyed.

For instance, you may no longer have the desire or drive to see your friends, perform your hobbies or participate in any recreational sports that you were doing before you started to notice overtraining occurring.

Essentially those who are verging on overtrained simply show very little desire to engage in life. Instead, they'd rather sit on the couch all day and sleep or just relax. Your body is trying to get you to rest by causing this fatigue so when this is the situation at hand, it's best to listen to it.

Increased Occurrence Of Infection or Illness

When you are constantly placing that high amount of stress on the body from your regular workouts, this is going to eventually begin to wear on your immune system.

Each and every day your body is going to get taxed – not only from your workout sessions but also from anything else that you encounter on a regular basis.

When either of these sources gets to be too much, the body will slowly begin to shut down. Since the immune system is what is responsible for dealing with all these stressors, when the stress gets to be too large, it's the one that is impacted.

As such, you're going to notice that you start becoming sick a lot more often or may even suffer from recurring infections that need medical treatment.

Overtraining is definitely going to impact you on more than just a muscular and athletic performance level and this fact illustrates this.

Cessation of Menstrual Cycle (for women)

Finally, if you're a woman and are verging on the edge of overtraining, one thing that may occur is that you actually lose your menstrual cycle. When you're working out very hard, especially if you happen to be eating a reduced calorie diet in order to promote fat loss, the body is going to start sensing this fuel shortage and begin to adapt.

Since reproduction consumes a large amount of energy by the body, it's going to do its best to prevent this from happening. The best way of doing that is to simply stop the menstrual cycle.

Women who are training many hours per week and burning up a great deal of calories will without a doubt have this fuel shortage (unless they are also eating a higher calorie diet) so if you see this occurring, it's your first sign you're doing too much.

Also, if this does occur, it's vital that you take action immediately and see your doctor as going without your monthly cycle can really put you at a higher risk of developing osteoporosis.

So there you have the main factors that you should be watching out for as you go about your workout program. When you're working with our trainers at End Result Fitness, all of this will be monitored and since the program itself is very planned out to ensure you aren't doing too much volume, the development of overtraining is very unlikely to occur.

Even still it's important that you're taking the time to talk with your trainer about how you're feeling as you go about your program and any issues that you may want to discuss.

This constant feedback and open discussion is vital to success and part of the ongoing effort to get you the *end result* you're looking for.

Now let's briefly go over what needs to be done should overtraining begin to present itself.

One Mandatory Week Off

The very first thing that you'll want to do should you notice overtraining starting to appear is take one week off. And by off, this means no cardio training, no weight training – just rest.

Some very light leisure activity can be performed just to get you off the couch and out, but keep in mind this is simply for movement purposes. You're not striving to burn calories nor are you striving to improve your fitness level.

Right now the body needs an extended period of rest and that's what you're going to focus on giving it.

High-Carb Feeding

Second, the next step in getting past the overtraining issue is to have one or sometimes even four or five high carb days in a row. Low carb diets naturally will tend to increase the risk of overtraining because of the fact that carbohydrates are what will be stored as muscle glycogen and when muscle glycogen is depleted, that's when higher levels of fatigue will be far more likely.

By having that high carb day or two while you're resting, you're going to restore the muscle glycogen levels and quite possibly also boost the metabolic rate.

Low carb diets also by nature tend to cause the body to slow its metabolic rate as it conserves calories so by adding the carbs back into the diet you boost it up again. This will come in especially handy when you're looking for fat loss as then when you move back on to your lower calorie diet again, fat loss continues to progress along.

Assessment Of Lifestyle Stress

Third, another important thing to do is to take a good look at your overall lifestyle as well. Remember, it isn't just workout stress that's going to impact your chances of overtraining. If you're extremely stressed out on a daily basis because of your job, relationships, or some other factor, when you add this stress to the stress of the workout, then it's far more likely to be more than the body can handle, thus overtraining sets in.

If, on the other hand, you lead a relatively low-stress lifestyle, then your body is mostly only going to have to deal with the stress from the workout session which is a lot more tolerable to take care of on a daily basis.

Look for areas of your life that are contributing high amounts of stress and see if there isn't a way you can control these better. It will definitely take some effort on your part to find better ways of dealing with this stress but the effort will be well worth it.

In the best case scenario you will just eliminate the stressor entirely from your lifestyle but if that's not going to be possible, then you'll want to consider looking at your coping methods and see if there isn't something you can do better to combat the build-up of stress.

Be sure that you talk to your trainer at End Result Fitness as well if stress is something that you're currently battling as we can help you find productive coping methods and healthier ways of dealing with it.

Re-Development Of Your Workout Program

Now that you've addressed the issue of actual overtraining, it's time to also take into account what you should be doing to make sure it doesn't happen again.

Step one is to make sure that you look at the overall structure of your workout. If you're doing too much volume per workout, too many sessions per week, or have some other structural issue with the program in general, this must get regulated.

Usually, this is the point when many people may consult a trainer at End Result Fitness to help them on their way as they aren't able to effectively determine just how much volume their body can handle total.

RE-Development Of Your Diet Program

Finally, the last thing to check out is what your diet program actually looks like. If you're not taking in enough calories to even come close to supporting your calorie needs (such as when you're doing a very intense workout program) that's going to create problems and will definitely set you up to experience overtraining syndrome.

Making sure you're getting enough calories first and foremost will be vital and then after that you'll also want to look and make sure that you're taking in enough protein as well as carbohydrates. These two macronutrients in particular tend to be most important so it's vital that you consider them and integrate them in the right amounts into your diet plan.

So that wraps up the discussion of overtraining. Overtraining is definitely a very real thing that many people deal with and battle. Fortunately when you do train with us in the studio, all of this will be looked at to ensure that you're not going to be at risk.

Now we'll move on to our next topic and one that many of you are likely wondering about, cardio training.

CHAPTER 26:
TO DO CARDIO OR TO NOT DO CARDIO –
WHAT'S THE SOLUTION

If there's one thing that's very highly debated in the industry of fitness and especially when speaking in the realm of fat loss, cardio training is it.

You get those specific individuals (usually cardio enthusiasts) who firmly believe that if you want to lose fat, cardio is the way to go about getting the job done.

These people hop onto the treadmill, bike, or the elliptical, day after day thinking that each workout is getting them closer to their goals.

But, often it doesn't. This is something that speaks for itself.

Then you have the second camp of people (usually the trainers) and they are the ones who know better. They're the ones who've seen the research and realize that cardio is simply an outdated technique for losing body fat.

They know that if you really are serious about getting to your goals, there are many things you should be doing and cardio just isn't one of them.

Now, this isn't to say all cardio is entirely bad. There are some specific types of cardio that can be beneficial but you must understand the pros and cons of it and then address the particular situation at hand.

That's what we're going to discuss next. First let's take a look at the various types of cardio that you can be doing so you can get a much better idea of what precisely this form of activity consists of.

Moderate Paced Steady State Cardio Training

The very first type of cardio and the most common that's being performed is your moderate paced steady state cardio training. This is the form of cardio where you go, hop onto the treadmill, and work at a steady pace for 30-60 minutes.

This kind of cardio is, quite frankly, boring.

Not only is it a drag to do but it's also not going to do a whole heck of a lot for your fitness level. It will burn off some calories (although at that moderate intensity it's not going to be burning off all that many) and it will help to increase your muscular endurance levels to an extent, but still, since it is only of moderate intensity, you aren't really pushing yourself all that hard so you can't expect to see great gains from this.

Remember that overloading stimulus principle – if you want to get stronger, faster, and more fit, you need to push the body past its comfort zone. That is what will get you the *end result* you're looking for.

Now, there are a few times when this steady state cardio training can come in somewhat handy. The first instance is when you are in need of cardio to do between two very intense workout sessions.

Since the body can only handle so much stress each week and weight lifting is a very stressful type of activity, if you're already verging on having enough total stress in the workout week, moderate paced cardio can be placed in without too much worry about overdoing this and moving into an overtrained state.

While if you're doing loads and loads of moderate paced cardio it will become too much of a stress on your system, for the most part if it's just one or two sessions a week added for heart health and to burn a few more calories, this generally doesn't prove to be a problem.

Moderate paced cardio workouts can be good for those who are doing four or five intense gym workouts as well.

Secondly, the next group of people who will benefit from moderate paced cardio workouts are those who are actually training for an endurance event.

If you're getting ready for a 5km, a 10km, a half marathon, or a full marathon, you'll obviously be adding the moderate paced cardio workouts into your week to help build up the volume tolerance you need to complete these events.

Interval Cardio Training

Moving on to the next form of cardio training. If you want to boost your level of fitness and really take your results up a notch, interval cardio training is going to be the way to go.

What this form of cardio training has you doing is alternating between bouts of very intense cardio activity for 20-60 seconds and then supplementing that with much lower levels of cardio intensity for 40-120 seconds (usually in a 1:2 or 1:3 work to rest ratio).

This form of training is by far the more effective form of cardio as far as fat burning is concerned. The reason for this is that while moderate paced cardio training will have you burning 5-10 calories per minute while you do it, interval training is going to help you increase the number of calories *after* the workout is finished.

After your moderate paced cardio session your metabolic rate returns back to normal, after a high intensity interval cardio training session you'll continue to burn calories over the course of the rest of the day.

All of these calories are really going to add up over the coming hours and over time this produces a very rapid rate of fat loss overall.

What's more is that since interval cardio training has you working at such a high intensity level, it's really going to challenge those muscle fibers to work harder than they've worked before and can actually be somewhat anabolic like a resistance training session would be.

Moderate paced cardio workouts on the other hand tend to be catabolic meaning they'll break down tissues in the body, and could eventually lead to a loss of lean muscle mass.

Since your muscle mass is the metabolic engine of the body – that is, the tissue that helps you burn the most calories while you sit around and do nothing, losing it should not be part of your game plan.

Finally, the last great thing about interval cardio training is that it's fast. You're in and out of the gym incredibly fast so this is perfect for those of you who have a very busy schedule.

Typically these are going to last somewhere between 15-20 minutes total with a warm-up and cool-down so they definitely won't take a huge time commitment on your part.

Now we come to the drawbacks however. The biggest drawback with this type of cardio training is the fact that it's going to be quite stressful on the nervous system so when you add that to your regular weight lifting workouts, you may find that it gets to be just a bit too much to keep up with.

Three or four weight lifting workouts a week as well as two to three interval cardio sessions a week is really going to be pushing the barrier and could set off that overtraining syndrome we talked about earlier.

Remember that your body does require rest each week (most effectively in the form of full days off) so getting yourself involved in too many sessions of interval cardio training as well as weight lifting is going to create numerous problems.

So there must be that balance. If you want to do more interval cardio workouts that's fine but just do be sure that you're also making note to reduce back slightly on the number of resistance training workouts you do as well in order to accommodate to that.

Resistance-Based Aerobic Conditioning

Now we move to the third form of cardio training, resistance based cardio training. This is the form that's starting to catch on more and more now as people are starting to look for ways to shorten their overall gym commitment time without having to sacrifice results.

This type of workout can do that. This is also the form of workout that's very often used when you work in studio with us because of the powerful fat burning benefits it has to offer. Not only will you get incredibly stronger while you do it but you're also going to improve your fitness level as well.

What you'll be doing in resistance based cardio training is performing a resistance based workout routine but keeping the overall pace up higher so that you're actually seeing cardio benefits as well.

This lets you then train both strength and cardio components of fitness all at once, literally cutting back your gym workout time by as much as half.

When doing this style of workout program, you'll be constantly moving from exercise to exercise and either alternating between strength based movements or adding in some cardio types activities. Pull-ups, burpees, squat jumps, walking lunges, push-ups, and ball crunches are all examples of exercises that you might perform while doing this type of workout set-up.

The great thing about this type of cardio too is that since the exercise is constantly changing (versus you staying in the same movement pattern as you would on some piece of cardio equipment) that in itself will help to promote greater progress levels since the body never knows what's happening next.

Furthermore, since you're doing strength based movements you'll also be hitting the agility and balance components of your fitness level as well really making for a well-rounded workout in general.

This really is a great way to go about designing your workout, particularly for those individuals who absolutely hate the traditional forms of cardio training and can help to build muscle mass and keep you nice and lean.

Recovery Cardio Training

Finally, we move on to our last form of cardio training which is recovery cardio training. This type of cardio training can literally be added at any point during the week and is just an incredibly light form of cardio training where you really won't be adding any additional stress to the body.

This type of cardio is mostly designed to help improve your overall recovery rates from your workouts but loosening up the muscle tissues, increasing blood flow to the region, and reducing any post workout soreness or inflammation that may be present.

With recovery cardio sessions, intensity is the last thing you're looking for as your general aim is to go at an incredibly light pace that has you hardly even getting your heart rate up.

Walking around the park, going for a leisurely bike ride, or going for a casual swim would all be considered recovery cardio sessions.

These can be done either later on in the day after your harder workout session is completed or done on off days between workout sessions. Listen to your body and do it whenever you feel like you need it.

Some people who do really experience quite a bit of post-workout soreness will find this cardio to be a lot more helpful than others. Listen to your body and judge how much you need based on how you're feeling.

Recovery cardio isn't going to interfere with your ability to rest up between sessions provided you're doing it correctly since it is – recovery cardio.

Choosing Your Ideal Cardio – Your How To Guide

So this may now leave you wondering what type of cardio you should be doing. First, you're going to have to assess your ability level. Obviously someone who's new to working out and isn't in the high level of shape that's necessary for interval sprints won't be able to dive into this type of cardio.

You'll have to work on developing that cardio base and then eventually bringing it up to that level as you can. Likewise, someone who's just learning the basic movements of resistance training won't be able to go from one exercise to the next the whole way through the workout without suffering from poor form as well as discouragement as they move along.

When you sit down with a trainer at End Result Fitness, you'll be discussing where you're at right now, where you'd like to go, and the best path to get there.

Then the trainer will help you develop a program that's right for you based on your skill level. This may mean starting out at a lower intensity of cardio and then slowly integrating more interval style of sessions into the mix as time goes on.

Another thing to consider is your own knowledge about your recovery system. If you know for a fact that you don't recover very well from your workouts then this is also a good indication that you shouldn't be forcing yourself to do multiple interval cardio workouts each week as well as those weight lifting workouts each week.

When you first begin designing your program, if you're aware that you do take a while to recover after a workout, let your trainer know this. It'll save time and frustration as they are then able to target the workout program specifically to your abilities.

Remember too that you never have to stay with just a single type of cardio training. It's perfectly possible to blend the types together throughout the workout week so that you can integrate them all into your routine.

Generally this works best as well since it will allow you to keep up your fitness level without risking overtraining. You may only do a single interval cardio session a week since you have a couple of circuit style workout programs and then to this also add a moderate paced cardio workout for endurance benefits.

Whatever your choice, always assessing your progress, your current goals, and your time availability will help ensure that you stay on track with where you need to be.

Just be sure that you're always watching out for that overtraining syndrome as it can creep up on you, especially if you are doing numerous cardio workouts.

Far too many people make that mistake of just thinking that they need to monitor their lifting sessions and that cardio won't influence how well they recover.

Not so. Cardio is still a stress on the body – granted, as we went over, different types of cardio place different stresses on the body, but it's a stress none-the-less and if you aren't taking it into account with the big picture, you're asking for trouble.

Cardio, while not the most effective form of activity for improving your body and fitness level, it is still important for overall good health purposes. It should always be incorporated into your workout routine in some regard.

You definitely do not need to spend hours doing it like many of you may be doing right now but it's definitely worth having a few sessions throughout the week to improve your heart health, enhance circulation, increase your muscular endurance, and get that positive endorphin release in the body that's going to put you in a good mood and feeling great!

Now, we're going to move on from our discussion of cardio training and talk about workouts on the go. For any of you who have trouble going to the gym regularly, this is a section you're really going to want to sit up and pay attention to. You will can learn how to deal with your busy schedule that keeps you away from the gym without it meaning abandoning your health and fitness goals.

CHAPTER 27:
WORKOUTS-TO-GO: STAY FIT WHILE TRAVELLING

Whether it's a business trip that's going to be keeping you out of the gym or your leisure vacation that you've been looking forward to for a number of months now, just because you're leaving the vicinity of your home gym does not mean you should take a break from your regular workout sessions.

This is going to be especially the case if you're often travelling for business because constantly stopping and restarting on your workout routine will leave progress far behind.

In order to see best results from any workout plan, continuality must be in place and if you're taking off one week every two, that's definitely not what's going on.

Fortunately, it's becoming easier and easier to stay in shape while on the road. As long as you plan for it, you should have no trouble maintaining your workout program.

Let's look at a few things that you should be doing right off the start in order to ensure your success.

1. Call Your Hotel

The very first thing you should always do is aim to book a hotel that offers a fitness facility.

As it will be a hotel gym often you can't really expect too much but if they have some basic cardio equipment and some dumbbells, this is definitely going to help you in your efforts.

When you have the equipment available to you this is one hurdle that you've just instantly overcome.

2. Schedule Your Sessions In

The second thing that you should be doing when travelling is making certain to schedule those workouts right into your day planner. If it's a leisure vacation this may not be as important as you'll typically have much more control of all the hours of the day, but if you're away on a business trip, plan a time before you get there for when you'll do your sessions.

Early morning typically always works best because you never know when work functions will run late or you'll get invited out to dinner or drinks with your colleagues. This then could easily push your workout entirely out of the way and cause you to lose focus.

Get it done first thing in the morning when you initially get up and then you can put it out of your mind knowing that you've done everything possible to keep up your fitness training.

3. Pack Any Equipment Needed

If the situation arises and you can't get into a hotel with a gym or you would prefer to stay in your room for your workout, then you need to consider some alternate options.

This is where resistance bands can come in incredibly handy since they are ultra light-weight and can easily be packed right into your suite case for use.

You can do almost any exercise with resistance bands to target all the main muscle groups so you shouldn't have any problem whatsoever coming up with something to do.

As long as you are willing to get creative, there are plenty of ways to fully challenge and stimulate the muscles.

Note that if you are someone who does have quite a bit of strength behind you (say a male who has been training for numerous years already), then you may need to double up on the resistance bands as you move throughout your workout.

This literally multiplies the amount of tension that will be placed upon the muscles throughout that workout thus boosting the overall intensity from the workout and will help you see the results you're looking for.

If you wish to bring any smaller ankle weights or something of that nature also consider that as it can add more challenge while doing a hotel room workout.

If you do happen to have an exercise ball that's very easy to inflate/deflate then definitely bring that since adding an exercise ball to the workout is a very excellent way to fully engage the core muscles more and increase the stress placed on the muscle tissues.

Remember that during your time away travelling from your usual workout program, your goal typically isn't to make extreme gains in progress but rather to maintain the current level you're at.

It can be quite beneficial in fact to periodize your program (focus on specific elements of fitness over the course of many months) so that during the time when you'll be travelling, that's actually designed active rest time.

This would then mean that the workouts are actually supposed to be of lower intensity and that the whole point during this time is to allow the body a bit more time to relax and recoup.

This way when you get back home again and hit those workouts hard, you're going to find that you're feeling fresh and full of energy, ready to go.

When on vacation, it can be especially a good time to really relax and help distress yourself, allowing you to reduce the risk of overtraining development.

4. Make A Few Modifications With Your Diet

Possibly the greatest concern while away travelling – even more than sticking with your workouts is maintaining some form of good dietary adherence.

While you may miss out on a few hundred calories burned if you don't do one of your schedule workouts, with some poor food choices it's very easy to consume 500-1000 calories over what you should be eating. If you're gone for a full week this could very easily cause a 1-2 pound body fat gain and that will set you back in your progress.

Your smartest strategy when it comes to your diet while you're away travelling is to consider first bringing as much healthy foods as you can with you to prepare as many meals and snacks as possible (or alternatively pick up some foods from a local grocery store and get a room with a kitchenette) and then designate just one or two meals each day where you will eat out.

At least then you only risk going over your calorie budget on those two meals and all the rest will stay constant.

Then, when out on those meals, always try and make the wisest choices possible. Remember that you generally can't go wrong with a grilled chicken breast with some steamed vegetable as long as you request it to be made without butter or oil and this is something that most restaurants can prepare.

If you're eating fast food, go with a salad with grilled chicken on top and request light dressing only and have it on the side.

There are plenty of ways to overcome the typical high calorie dishes of most restaurants as long as you are willing to make some wise adjustments.

Drinking is always something that tends to come up whether you're away on business or away on vacation and you should aim to avoid it as much as possible.

Remember that alcohol will contain empty calories and will slow down the rate of fat loss (which we'll be getting into in more details in a coming chapter).

Obviously, if you're on vacation and want to indulge in a few alcohol drinks then chances are you're going to do so but at the very least if you can keep it to a somewhat minimum and make sure that the mixers you're adding are all low in calories you shouldn't see too much damage being done.

Remember moderation is the most important thing to always remember when on vacation when it comes to both alcohol intake as well as the foods you're ordering as if you do practice it, the damage will always be minimal.

Try and avoid that 'all or none' thinking process that some people get into where if they blow it just a little bit, they might as well blow it big time.

A few extra calories at a meal will hardly put a dent in your fat loss plan but if you have those few extra hundred calories and then figure all hope is lost and proceed to take in an extra thousand calories, now you've really outdone yourself.

Don't let yourself get too frustrated if you aren't 100% perfect while away and remember to take each day and meal at a time.

If you stay in this frame of mind the chances that you stay in control of your choices and don't let one little mistake get the best of you will be that much greater.

There you have some of the top tips for maintaining your fitness while travelling. If you're someone who goes away from home only once or twice a year, it's really not going to make that big of a difference what you do – it's such a small frame of time when you look at the bigger picture of things that you can easily make up for a bit of damage the rest of the time.

But, if you're travelling at least once a month or more frequently, you must get on top of this game. Otherwise, all your time back is going to be spent undoing the damage from the time away and you're never going to make any progress forwards.

Now let's move on and talk about another issue that can hamper your fitness goals – a lack of time. This is something that most of you will be dealing with so it's another topic to pay close attention to.

CHAPTER 28:
TIME PRESSED WORKOUT SOLUTION

At some point or another, a very common issue that you're going to run into is a lack of time. Many of us have the best intensions of doing the workout so it's definitely not a factor of being too lazy to go to the gym, but rather, it's a matter of life just being way too busy.

Sometimes, as important as your workouts are, other things become the priority.

When this occurs, does it mean you have to forgo your health and fitness goals? Certainly not. In fact, if you are smart about how you handle this situation, you can still see great gains in progress without having to devote hours to the gym each week.

The key thing to always remember when it comes to fitting in workouts when you're short in time is that you want to make them as intense as possible.

Intensity will beat out duration any day of the week anyway, so you may actually be doing yourself a favour by squeezing your workout into that short time span.

Some of us do have a habit of taking a more leisurely pace about our normal workouts, which will directly influence how hard your body is working, but when you're pressed for time and trying to get in what you need to in 15-20 minutes, all of a sudden, 'leisurely' isn't a word that's in your vocabulary. You're in the gym fighting to make the most out of every minute you've got.

Now, the best case scenario is always going to be if you can aim to still keep up your workouts with your trainer at End Result Fitness. Even if it is just one session a week, that will ensure that you keep moving forward.

Talk with your trainer about the lack of time in your life and you will both be able to come up with a solution together.

Right now we're going to go over some of the best methods to use to help cut back the total time of your workouts so you can make the most of what little time you do have. Again, many of these will be integrated into your workouts with your trainer during that time, so this is more for you to keep in mind in any workouts you may do outside of your sessions with End Result Fitness.

Some of you will be doing a few sessions on your own while others will be working pretty much exclusively with a trainer. This all depends on what package you sign up for and what you feel is right for your individual situation.

Let's show you the methods.

Focus On Strictly Compound Movements

The very first thing that you must be doing if you're pressed for time is making certain to only be performing compound movements. At this point you really don't have time to be doing isolation exercises that are just going to offer way too little pay-off for you to invest your time into them.

Instead, look to the movements that will target multiple areas of the body. If you can hit three muscle groups at once rather than one, you're one step ahead of the gym.

This means fewer exercises total per workout meaning you get in, get your workout done, and get out very quickly.

As we touched upon earlier, these are the exercises that are going to have you burning up the most calories as well so by doing them, you move closer to your end goal of seeing rapid fat loss taking place.

Superset Your Exercises

Second, another very effective technique that you'll definitely want to use as you progress throughout your program is to superset your exercises. This is used very often in advanced program plans to boost the intensity of the overall workout but during a time pressed workout, it's also one method that you'll want to be putting to good use.

Since it has you doing two exercises immediately back to back with no rest in between, that's really going to cut down on the total time you spend doing the workout.

When pressed for time like this, the best option here will be to superset an upper body exercise together with a lower body exercise. While doing both upper body or both lower body exercises is definitely a good way to go about doing supersets as well, the drawback with that is that you will likely need longer to rest between the superset of two of the similar muscle groups.

Since your upper body will rest entirely while you're doing your lower body exercise and vice versa, this further allows you to keep up the pace of the overall workout as 30 seconds rest should likely be enough.

The goal here is to cut back on all time spent resting so you can get through your workout as fast as possible and this will accomplish that goal nicely.

Add Cardio Intervals Between Strength Moves

Third, another idea if you're someone who's only hitting the gym two or three days a week and therefore needs to accomplish both cardiovascular training as well as strength training in the same session is to add some cardio intervals in between your strength moves.

This does tend to work best with upper body exercises as doing a minute sprint between sets of squats for example would be a sheer brutality.

If you do an upper body exercise though and then move over to the treadmill to do your sprint, since your lower body is feeling fairly fresh still so the overall progress will not be nearly as limited.

Or, another way to go about this so that you can incorporate some lower body exercises into the mix is to perform a lower body exercise, an upper body exercise, and then do your cardio interval. Finally, rest after all that's completed for 30 seconds to one minute and then repeat through once again.

However you want to set it up should work well and even if you decide against doing the cardio training in there, don't think that you won't still get some cardiovascular conditioning benefits from the supersets themselves.

Since you are keeping up that quick pace, the heart will definitely be working to move through your resistance based movements and that in itself will definitely bring you some benefits.

Perform Full Body Workouts

Finally, our last point for time-pressed workout solutions is to really consider a full body approach. Unless your situation is that you can get to the gym daily but only have a very limited time span, full body workouts are going to ensure that you keep up the overall training frequency (which is very important for best results) with that low time commitment.

The minimum number of times each muscle in your body should get worked will be twice, so two, 30 minute full body workouts isn't really too much to ask for. Make it one, as long as you keep up that minimum of one training session with your trainer at End Result Fitness.

This leaves plenty of free days up in your week to do all the other activities and obligations you have to tend to without having to let it sacrifice your fitness goals.

Or, going back to the other scenario, if you can make it to the gym more frequently, then you could do the upper/lower workout set-up. If you break the body in half like this, it means there are fewer muscle groups you have to target so once again, less overall time being devoted to that session. But this set-up will require four sessions each week so you must have that type of availability for it to work.

There you have all the main concepts to remember for short workout solutions.

Next up on our discussion list is the concept of active rest and why this is important.

CHAPTER 29:
ACTIVE REST – WHY IT'S A MUST

When you're very intensely focused on losing body fat, firming and defining your muscles, and moving closer to your end goal, rest seems like the last thing you should be doing.

You have a goal to reach and there's work to be done! – at least that's what you're likely thinking.

But the one thing that some people fail to take into account is the fact that if you're not providing enough rest between your workout sessions and from week to week, you're actually doing yourself a huge disservice.

When you train with us at End Result Fitness, we are dedicated to getting you to your *end result* and as such, will integrate rest days right into your routine.

If you're currently using a workout routine that does not allow for this time off, that's your very first signal that something's not right with your plan.

Think of it like this. Each time you go into the gym and hit those muscles, you're creating tiny tears within their structure. After the workout's done, you're actually much weaker than when you went into the gym – which you've very likely noticed before.

At the start of the workout lifting those 20 pound dumbbells may not have felt too bad but if you were to attempt a lift at the very end, 10 pounds may be enough of a challenge.

Your body is tired, broken down, and crying for rest.

Then once you're finished the workout period, the body immediately goes into a high recovery period where it rapidly begins repairing all those broken down muscle tissues.

Assuming you provide good nutrition, this process takes place rather quickly and you build yourself back up to where you were before only a little bit stronger now (since the body wants to ensure it isn't as worn out if it encounters that stress again at a later time).

The harder and more demanding your workout is at this point, the longer that recovery is going to take. While it is 'rapid' in the sense that the time period immediately after the workout is critical for overall results, it's not so rapid that you could go back to the gym later on in the day and hit the muscles again.

Generally, the best rule to follow is to give each muscle tissue at least 48 hours of rest between workout sessions. This gives you two full night's to recover (sleep is also 'prime time' as far as recovery is concerned).

The problem some people experience when their workout is not well designed is that they will place two workouts back to back that they think are working different muscle groups but really those same muscles are still working indirectly. This will quickly be changed when they begin working with End Result Fitness.

Remember, when you perform those compound exercises you're working multiple muscle groups all at once. So even though you may think you're primarily working the chest when you do a bench press or a push-up, you're still also hitting the triceps as well.

As such, doing shoulder presses the next day (where triceps are also targeted) wouldn't be a wise decision.

This is also why full body or upper/lower splits are so good – since that rest day is built in, you'll naturally overcome this issue.

This also doesn't take into account CNS fatigue as well, which is very predominant and must be considered. If you're in the gym lifting weights day in and day out, you're really taxing your CNS. Eventually it will become too much and even though your muscles may be recovering, your central nervous system isn't and you burn out.

It's definitely not the situation you want to find yourself in.

That's where active rest comes into play. Many of you aren't going to want to be taking numerous days off each week since you do have goals to reach, like we mentioned above, so by adding in active rest days, you'll help relieve your desire to exercise without reducing your rate of recovery.

What is active rest?

Essentially it's any type of exercise that's performed at a much lower intensity that your body can easily tolerate.

A brisk walk around your neighbourhood, a family bike ride through the park, a day spent outside doing some gardening; these would also count as active rest.

Yes, you are moving around and being active, but you're not overloading the muscles in any way or adding a higher degree of overall stress.

Rest and recovery can still take place without you having to plant yourself on the couch for a full day straight.

Most people find that this active rest is actually going to boost their recovery because it gets the blood flowing to the muscle tissues and will reduce the build-up of lactic acid.

Since that's the stuff that tends to make you very sore after a workout, anything you can do to reduce it will definitely come in helpful.

In most workout programs, one to two days should be devoted to active rest, which will still leave plenty of time left for your intense workout sessions that get you to your *end result*.

Now, the above all described active rest as a means to speed recovery, you also do have another form of rest that is slightly more passive, but still offers numerous health benefits.

These are *relaxation* based exercises that will help to tone down your overall stress levels, improving how well you recover from your workout sessions.

Remember that stress in general – be it workout stress, work stress, or any other type of stress, hampers your recovery. It's going to tax your immune system and make the process move along that much more slowly.

Doing what you can to take care of this stress build-up will result in faster progress from your workout sessions, again moving you closer to your *end result*.

Great relaxation based activities that you'll want to consider adding to the program include things like yoga, meditation, or tai chi. These will focus on improving the breathing patterns, increasing blood flow throughout the body, relaxing the tired muscles, and putting you in an all around better frame of mind.

These types of workouts will also not interfere with your usual intense workout sessions either, so they are easily added into any workout routine you may be doing.

Obviously, you're still going to have to find the time to get these activities in, but even dedicating yourself to doing just one per week can make a difference. If you feel less stressed out because of it, make no mistake, it is well worth your time.

Now that covers all the informatoin you need to know to get you from where you are now to your *end result*. With our help you can definitely achieve the look you're going for and won't have to spend hours and hours in the gym like some of you may have thought before.

In fact, with the right type of training, making significant changes in your body takes just a few hours a week along with some smart dietary strategies. You will be amazed at the type of results that you can get.

Now let's move on and get to your workout program samples.

CHAPTER 30:
YOUR WORKOUT PROGRAMS

The following are some great guidelines for you to follow for workouts that you can do from the comfort of your home and many of which will be referred to by the trainer that you work with at End Result Fitness.

This is an excellent place for anyone to start to build up a nice level of fitness upon which you'll build on when you start working with your trainer at End Result Fitness. When working in studio, each of these workouts will get further customized to your own individual needs so you can be sure that you're seeing the absolute best results possible.

Generally, how many of these workouts you'll be completing will depend on how many times you're seeing your trainer in the studio. If you're working with us 4 times a week, only a few cardio sessions may be necessary while if you're just seeing us in studio twice a week, then your trainer may advise you to do a few of the workouts on the next few pages as well.

You'll find that all of the resistance based workouts take less than 30 minutes to complete so these are designed with a busy lifestyle in mind. We understand that you won't have hours each day to dedicate to your fitness program and we still promote that you will be able to get to that *end result* without having to put in massive amounts of time.

The workouts are fast paced, focused on intensity, and will work all the muscles in the body so you won't have to worry about developing any type of muscular imbalances. This is a critical factor of any workout as well as it's what will keep you injury free in the long run.

For the workouts you'll require very minimal equipment as well so most of you should easily be able to do these in the comfort of your own home. If you can get a stability and medicine ball, a set of adjustable dumbbells with enough weight that you're going to feel fully challenged, as well as an adjustable bench, you'll be all set.

On the next few pages, you'll see both the beginner as well as the intermediate program listings. These are best done in conjunction with the workouts your trainer gives you and when you speak to your End Result Fitness trainer in the studio they will be instructing you on which workouts you'll be performing.

Note that once you get past the intermediate stage level, that's when you're definitely going to want to be consulting with a trainer and not going at this alone. There will be many advanced strategies to be using and if you don't have them implemented properly, the chances of injury and burnout are much higher.

Beginner's 3 Day A Week Full Body Workout Program

You are to perform two sets of each superset taking just 30 to 60 seconds of rest in between each one. Also note that if you would like, you can add in an ab exercise as listed as 'active recovery' between each superset you do.

This will not only help keep your heart rate at a more reasonable level but also help to boost your metabolic rate over the course of the entire workout session.

Day 1:

Superset #1:

Dumbbell Chest Press – 12-15 reps
Dumbbell Squats – 12-15 reps

Optional Ab Exercise: Crunches on an Exercise Ball

Superset #2:

Bent Over Dumbbell Rows – 12-15 reps
Lunges – 12-15 reps

Optional Ab Exercise: Lying Leg Raises

Superset #3:

Dumbbell Shoulder Press – 12-15 reps
Dumbbell Pull-Overs – 12-15 reps

Optional Ab Exercise: Plank – 30 seconds hold

Day 2:

Superset #1:

Incline Chest Press – 12-15 reps
Dumbbell Sumo Squats – 12-15 reps

Optional Ab Exercise: Crunches on an Exercise Ball

Superset #2:

Bent Over 1-Arm Dumbbell Rows – 12-15 reps
Step-Ups – 12-15 reps

Optional Ab Exercise: Lying Leg Raises

Superset #3:

Dumbbell Shoulder Press on an Exercise Ball – 12-15 reps
Jump Squats – 12-15 reps

Optional Ab Exercise: The Bicycle

Day 3:

Superset #1:

Chest Press on an Exercise Ball – 12-15 reps
Exercise Ball Wall Squats – 12-15 reps

Optional Ab Exercise: Lying Leg Raises

Superset #2:

Bent Over Dumbbell Rows – 12-15 reps
Reverse Dumbbell Lunges – 12-15 reps

Optional Ab Exercise: The Plank – 30 seconds hold

Superset #3:

Dumbbell Shoulder Press – 12-15 reps
Walking Dumbbell Lunges – 12-15 reps

Optional Ab Exercise: Side Crunches on an Exercise Ball

Beginner's Core/Abs Workout

Perform each exercise for 12-15 reps, trying to progress throughout the workout as quickly as possible. Repeat the entire cycle of exercises twice for best results.

Crunches on an Exercise Ball
Lying Leg Raises
Plank (30 second hold)
Bicycle Exercise
Lying Back Raises
Plank (30 second hold)

Intermediate 3 Day A Week Full Body Program

You are to perform three sets of each superset taking just 30 to 60 seconds of rest in between each one. Also note that if you would like you can add in an ab exercise as listed as 'active recovery' between each superset you do.

This will not only help keep your heart rate at a more reasonable level but also help to boost your metabolic rate over the course of the entire workout session.

Day 1:

Superset #1:

Dumbbell Squats – 12-15 reps
Dumbbell Chest Press – 12-15 reps
Dumbbell Bent Over Rows – 12-15 reps
Dumbbell Bicep Curls – 12-15 reps

Optional Ab Exercise: Crunches on an Exercise Ball

Superset #2:

Dumbbell Lunges – 12-15 reps
Dumbbell Shoulder Press – 12-15 reps
Dumbbell Step-Ups – 12-15 reps
Dumbbell Bent Over Tricep Extension – 12-15 reps

Optional Ab Exercise: Crunches on an Exercise Ball

Day 2:

Dumbbell Stiff Legged Deadlifts – 12-15 reps
Dumbbell Chest Press on an Exercise Ball – 12-15 reps
Dumbbell Bent Over Rows – 12-15 reps
Dumbbell Lateral Raises Sitting on an Exercise Ball – 12-15 reps

Optional Ab Exercise: Prone Ball Roll Ins

Superset #2:

Dumbbell Reverse Lunges – 12-15 reps
Dumbbell Shoulder Press – 12-15 reps
Dumbbell Squats – 12-15 reps
Dumbbell Front Raises Sitting on an Exercise Ball– 12-15 reps

Optional Ab Exercise: Crunches on an Exercise Ball

Day 3:

Superset #1:

Jump Squats – 12-15 reps
Push-Ups – 12-15 reps
Dumbbell Shoulder Press – 12-15 reps
Dumbbell Bicep Curls – 12-15 reps

Optional Ab Exercise: Side Crunches on A\an Exercise Ball

Superset #2:

Dumbbell Sumo Squats – 12-15 reps
Dumbbell Incline Chest Press – 12-15 reps
Dumbbell Bent Over Rows – 12-15 reps
Dumbbell Overhead Tricep Extensions - 12-15 reps

Optional Ab Exercise: Plank on an Exercise Ball

Intermediate Core/Abs Workout

Perform each exercise for 12-15 reps, trying to progress throughout the workout as quickly as possible. Repeat the entire cycle of exercises three times through for best results.

Prone Ball Roll Ins
Crunches on an Exercise Ball
Lying Leg Raise
Plank on an Exercise Ball (one minute hold)
Side Crunches on an Exercise Ball
Russian Twists on an Exercise Ball
V-Sit ups
Plank on an Exercise Ball (one minute hold)

Cardio Workouts

Now we move on to the cardio workout side of things. When you meet up with your trainer, they will also instruct you on how many cardio workouts you'll be doing but refer to this handy guide for reference so you know what they are referring to when they name a specific workout.

Fat Burning Cardio

Your fat burning cardio sessions are designed to up the intensity as much as possible while boosting your overall level of fitness.

For these, you are to choose a mode of cardio that you enjoy – running is by far the best option if you can do it and alternate between all out, 100% effort sprints with active rest intervals where you work at a much, much lower intensity level.

When you work in studio with an End Result Fitness trainer you will use a tool called the Jacobs ladder which proves to be even more effective than running, so that's another thing to look forward to when doing your sessions there.

So the set-up will look something like this:
(where RPE = rate of perceived exertion)

5 minute warm-up

30 seconds RPE 8
60 seconds RPE 3
30 seconds RPE 9
60 seconds RPE 3
30 seconds RPE 10
60 seconds RPE 3
30 seconds RPE 9
60 seconds RPE 3
30 seconds RPE 8
60 seconds RPE 3

5 minute cool-down

Slow and Steady Fat Melting Cardio

The second cardio option that your End Result Trainer may refer to is the slow and steady fat melting cardio option.

This type of cardio is best performed first thing in the morning on an empty stomach if possible or on the off days from your regular training.

Since it's not quite as intense on the body as the interval cardio style is you'll find that you recover much more quickly from it and it doesn't take quite as much out of you.

The goal here is to maintain your aerobic fitness while working on this form of cardio as well as increase your daily calorie burn.

Here's what this set-up may look like:

5 minute warm-up

30-45 minutes at RPE 6-8

5 minute cool-down

It's simple and straightforward. If you can, aim to select a different piece of fitness equipment each time you're doing it so that you don't get bored and likewise, your body never gets used to just one form of activity.

SECTION 4:
BUILDING A FAT LOSS AND WEIGHT MAINTENANCE LIFESTYLE

Now that you've seen just what it takes to put together a very successful fat loss program, it's time to start looking at what it takes to make this a *lifestyle* change. If you want to see nothing but the best of results from your program, this needs to be something that you're going to fully commit to 100% and carry it out every step of the way.

If you approach any type of program with a 'quick-fix' solution in mind and don't intend to make actual lifestyle changes that are going to help you maintain the results you've seen and possibly even improve your fitness level further, you're never going to see long-term success.

The real fat loss winners are those who are able to maintain their weight loss for more than six consecutive months because by that point, positive habits have been formed and they are very likely well on their way to keeping that weight off forever.

What we're going to go over now are some of the top tricks of the trade that you can use to help you maintain your healthy diet and continue to look your best.

Keep in mind that each and every one of you will likely come up with a few of your own methods as well. Motivation is a very personal thing and what motivates one person to keep up their diet and workouts could do absolutely nothing for another.

By learning your own individual preferences and what inspires you to keep going you're giving your best every step of the way. What is important though is that even though you have reached the goals you set for yourself at this moment, you don't let yourself become complacent.

Set some new goals – go after a new workout objective or shift the focus over to athletic goals instead of body composition goals.

One way to ensure that you are keeping yourself in check is to never go without a goal. Whether it's workout performance goals, bodyweight goals, or some other goal that you want to achieve, having something that you are actively working towards is going to be the first step to keeping up with your program.

It's when we don't have any form of direction in place that most people will quickly fall off the bandwagon because at that point there's no driving force.

Who cares if you miss a workout? It's not like it's going to impact anything?

You have no goal.

But, if you do have a goal, then too many skipped workouts is going to mean missing out on your deadline (as always, be sure that these are *smart* goals that you're setting).

Having those goals in place will do wonders for your motivational level so never try and go without. That's one of the top pieces of advice for long-term adherence and success.

Since most people are very motivated by a sense of achievement, when you have that goal you're working towards, achievement will be yours.

Let's get right to it and first begin discussing some of the tricks that you can use to help stick with your diet.

As you've already seen, diet is at least 50% of the weight maintenance game so it's important that you don't ever let yourself detour too far off course.

CHAPTER 31:
TOOLS AND TECHNIQUES FOR STICKING WITH YOUR DIET

By far, sticking with a healthy diet is the one thing that most of us struggle with. This is partly due to the pleasure factor. For most people, food is a huge source of pleasure and something we just aren't quite willing to do away with.

Hopefully, by this point you've taken some time to experiment with various food prep techniques so you've created a few healthier meals that do taste great.

If you can get creative in the kitchen, that's definitely going to be one of the best ways to help yourself maintain the diet plan.

Below are a few other quick methods that you can use. Most people can find the time to exercise at some point in their week but saying no too foods that seem to be really calling their name is a whole other story.

These techniques can help.

Pre-Plan Your Meals

One of the largest reasons many people will stray from their diet is simply an issue of not pre-planning their meals. They don't know what they're eating for lunch when they get up in the morning and thus leave it to chance.

Remember, anything left to chance is likely to end up far less healthier than you would like. It simply is not that easy to find incredibly healthy food on the go so if you aren't planning your meals out, you're basically leaving your body weight maintenance up to chance as well.

In the best case scenario, you should always aim to sit down every Sunday evening and plan out all your meals for the coming week. This way, there's no question of what's for dinner and no chance for take-out or that oven-bake pizza in the freezer to creep its way into your menu plan.

You have a set target in mind and won't have to think twice about it. Remember, those who fail to plan, plan to fail. It may be an overused saying but again in this case, it's 100% correct.

If you take time, you can usually have 100% control over your food intake. This will help out hugely when it comes to preventing fat gain.

If you can't take the time to plan out all your meals over the weekend, at least try and do it on a nightly basis. If nothing else, make a decision of what's for breakfast, lunch, and dinner.

Snacks are slightly easier to fill and a bit easier to also find healthier choices for but those main meals leave too much room for high-calorie foods to come into play.

Come up with a schedule for your healthy meals and do your best to stick with it.

Pre-Cook Your Meals

Now, if you really want to take being prepared to a whole new level, try and pre-cook as many of your meals ahead of time as you can.

Again on Sunday, once you have figured out what you'll be eating for the rest of the week, start to cook as much as you can of those meals at that point so that it's all ready to go throughout the week.

Lack of time is another big barrier for many people so if they're rushing off to some obligation they have in the evening, the chances of them grilling up some chicken, chopping some vegetables, and so on is just not that high.

Fortunately, there is plenty that can be done ahead of time.

First, be sure to cook up as much of your protein sources as you can. Chicken, beef, turkey, and salmon can all be prepared throughout the weekend and placed in the freezer for the coming week.

Then all you need to do is take the cooked protein out to let thaw the night before and you're all ready to go in that area of the meal.

Likewise, invest in some frozen vegetables to keep on hand at all times. These are easily tossed into a soup, stir-fry, or just boiled to have as a side dish. It beats the chopping that you'd have to do with fresh when you're in a rush.

Sure, fresh may taste slightly better to most people, but when you're pressed for time, frozen is definitely better than nothing. Just do be careful with canned vegetables however as even though it is a fast option, usually these are loaded with salt.

If you like, you can also consider freezing any cooked meals you may want to make as well. Stir-fry's, stews, soups, and casseroles are all easily frozen to eat throughout the week.

Having these quick meals on the go that you've prepared yourself can really be the saving grace when you want to stick with your diet plan.

Also, in addition to the cooking aspect of preparing the meals ahead of time, be sure that you do as much grocery shopping for the foods in those meals as well.

Having to run to the grocery store each day to pick up groceries is a real time killer so if you can aim to keep everything you need on hand before the week begins, you'll be all set.

Many of the wholesome staples you should have – brown rice, oatmeal, quinoa, barley, potatoes, egg whites, cottage cheese, frozen chicken breasts, natural nut butter, etc will last for weeks in the fridge so make it an aim to do a larger shopping trip once every two weeks or so to stock up so then if you do have to run to the store, it's only for smaller items that you can purchase quickly.

Come Up With Convenient Snacks

Another great quick tip that will help you maintain your meal plan is to come up with some quick convenient snack ideas as well. Many of us are quick to turn to the pre-packaged convenient snacks – energy bars, granola bars, rice chips, crackers, and so on which aren't really going to provide the wholesome nutrition that you're looking for.

Instead, aim to do your best to pick out a few classic stand-by's that you can turn to for snacks that you'll keep in your desk or car that won't wreck your diet.

For instance, trail mix made yourself is a great option that contains healthy carbs, fats, and some protein.

Likewise, a pop-top can of tuna along with some whole wheat crackers can also make for a good snack when your stomach is growling and you're stuck at work late.

For at home, always try and purchase pre-chopped fresh vegetables to have on hand that you can snack on when you want something to put in your mouth.

Or consider purchasing the lower sugar, low fat yogurt cups and serve those with a cup of berries for a sweet dessert to kill late night cravings.

When you have plenty of other options to turn to it really will reduce the chances that you decide to go for that bowl of Chunky Monkey in the freezer and totally set you a day back on your healthy eating plan.

Make It A Habit To Try New Recipes

Another good habit that's excellent to get into that will really save your nutrition plan is making sure that you regularly are trying out new recipes.

It's perfectly natural for anyone to get bored when they're eating the same foods over and over again so by constantly changing it up and trying out a new recipe, you'll prevent boredom from kicking in.

When you do this there's a much lower chance that you're going to experience those high food cravings and eventually move right away from the plan altogether.

There are so many recipes available that promote healthier eating so there's really no shortage of options here.

Whether you're using a very low carb diet plan or are on a more mixed approach aimed at adding more lean muscle mass to your frame, you really should have no trouble finding something to prepare for your meal.

Try and utilize a variety of different lower fat, lower calorie cooking methods as well such as steaming, stir-frying, baking, or grilling. Each of these will create a unique blend of flavours in the food and help up its appeal to your taste buds.

Don't Neglect Cheat Meals

Finally, the last thing that you must make sure you're going to do if you're going to have success with maintaining a healthy eating plan in the long-term is to make sure that you don't neglect regular cheat meals.

While you definitely do not want to give yourself too much slack here and start having cheat meals every second day, if you go too long without letting yourself indulge in foods you are craving, you could bring about a food binge, which could then lead to quite a bit of trouble.

The great thing about maintaining your weight loss in the long run is that now that the initial weight has been lost, you don't have to be quite as strict with your meal plan as you were before when you were losing the weight.

One method that many people use to maintain their weight which works quite well is to still eat relatively lower calorie throughout the week. When the weekend hits and they are out and about being more social and if they do happen to indulge a bit here and there, it doesn't hurt them too much and they still see great results.

Since it will be the total weekly calorie intake that makes the biggest difference of whether you gain or lose weight, if you can get it to where it needs to be overall, that's all that matters.

So someone may choose to consume 2000 calories per day for all seven days (a total of 14,000 calories overall for the week), or someone may choose to consume 1500 calories Monday through Friday and then have around 3000 calories on both Saturday and Sunday.

Both people would take in about the same amount of weekly calories so their weights would stay slightly similar.

It all depends on what you prefer. If you like more day to day flexibility and don't like feeling at all restricted, go for the nice even intake throughout the week.

On the other hand, if you're someone who really likes your cheat meals and wants to go out on the weekend and not worry about what you're eating as much, then choose the second strategy.

As long as you're longer term calorie intake adds up to where it needs to be, both strategies will work out very well.

The biggest thing to remember with your cheat meals is that if you do notice that you are starting to gain body weight it's time to immediately begin to cut back.

Getting the situation back under control right away is the absolute best game plan for maintaining your body weight in the long run. Take action if you see it get out of control and you'll only be dealing with the issue for a week at most.

That gives you a good number of ideas on how you can work to maintain your diet in the long term. Remember that just because you have lost the weight it does not mean it's now a free for all with your diet plan.

You still must maintain some degree of control otherwise you'll quickly slip right back into your old habits and once again be starting on a full blown weight loss plan.

Now let's go over to the workout side of things and give you some tips and techniques for helping to stick with that. Just like the diet, maintaining exercise over the long haul is very important for weight maintenance. It's what will help you keep a higher metabolic rate throughout the day, keep your body fat percentage lower, and keep your muscles and bones strong.

CHAPTER 32:
MAINTAINING WORKOUT MOTIVATION

As we discussed in the introduction to this section, making sure that you're constantly setting new goals for yourself is one of the best ways to maintain workout motivation and keep yourself pushing forwards.

Don't ever get too comfortable with your workouts because when you do, that's when you first stop seeing the results that you want and second, stop feeling interested in continually going to the gym itself.

Most of us in general need to have something that we're working towards so we get that feeling of self-betterment. When you don't have this, that's when motivation will really begin to dwindle.

Now let's take a look at a few other tips to consider that will help to boost your motivational level and get you sticking with those workout sessions.

Find A Workout Partner

One of the single best ways to maintain motivation for your workouts is to start working out with a partner. This is also a big reason why at End Result Fitness you'll always be training with someone else and your trainer.

By getting that other person involved you're adding a whole new social aspect to the workout which is something that does keep most people coming back for more.

Also, when you know that person is relying on you to show up for your workout, you're really going to think twice about skipping out of it as well.

It can be fun to come up with a small challenge between you and your workout partner as well to keep you both motivated and right on track. Set a small reward for whoever reaches their goal first and then agree on an intended deadline to reach those goals.

Make sure that you do have that deadline set however, as that will ensure that each of you holds the other accountable.

Make Your List Of Motivational Reasons

The second way to help motivate yourself to stick with a workout program is to make a list of all the reasons why you are doing this in the first place.

Sometimes as we get all wrapped up in our training sessions it can be easy to forget the primary purpose we got started in the first place.

By constantly reminding yourself what it is you're working towards, you can help increase the rate of success that you do achieve your *end result*.

Remember that it's always best to include a variety of different reasons from aesthetic reasons (such as looking better in that hot new pair of jeans you just purchased) to health reasons such as decreasing your blood pressure and boosting the amount of energy you have on a daily basis.

Or, perhaps you're looking for performance based results such as increasing your bench press ten pounds or decreasing your one mile run time.

Whatever your particular reasons are, list them out on a sheet of paper and put it somewhere that you'll see it daily.

Review it first thing in the morning when you wake up and last thing before you go to bed so it'll always be fresh in your mind whenever you need to call upon these when you're tempted to skip out on a workout session.

Use Pictures For Motivational Purposes

Another great strategy to enhance your motivation is to also start using some pictures as well. Since many people are very visual by nature, if you have pictures that you can look to that resemble what it is you want to look like once you've achieved your end goal, that too can push you along the path to success.

One thing that is very vital with these pictures is to ensure that they are something that you could realistically strive to reach. Don't get caught up finding a picture of your favorite celebrity with a size two waist when you know for a fact that you'd have to lose actual bone tissue to get that thin!

There are always going to be certain structural limitations that you could be facing with any type of transformation you want to complete. It's important that you do take time to realize that and take into account any adjustments in expectations that must be made.

While you should always strive to reach the best you can be, you need to understand what is realistic and what is not. Doing so is going to help you succeed that much faster.

In addition to finding pictures of what you *want* to look like, it can also be quite helpful to find pictures of what you *used* to look like. By this I'm referring to your before pictures that you took at the start. Look back on them now that you're progressing along and you'll see just how far you've come.

This is one of the biggest motivational strategies for many people because it allows them to realize how much progress they really are making in times when it feels as though they're making none.

While progress may be very slow at times, as long as it's *slow and steady*, that's what you're after here. Remember that you likely won't see day to day changes. Sometimes you may hardly notice a change week to week.

But, when you look back over the course of the month, that may be when it becomes very clear that you have in fact made some really great gains towards improving your progress.

Make Daily Challenges

The next way to help motivate yourself to stick with your workouts is to set little daily challenges for yourself.

We've already talked about the importance of having a long-term goal set along with numerous mini-goals along the way. You really can't do without these if you do hope to stick with your program in the long run because they are in a major way going to help fuel your desire to keep pushing onwards.

But sometimes those mini-goals aren't even enough. There are times when your motivational level is just really lagging behind and that smaller reward or goal just seems to be miles away.

Then what?

It's time to turn to daily challenges. These aren't really goals per say as they should be something that you could very realistically obtain in the here and now. Essentially something that you don't really have to work to obtain but more like just put in the work and they will come.

These challenges should push you further than you have in the past so you will definitely have to work at it, but it should be doable – now.

For instance, let's say last time you were in the gym you did a set of 8 on the shoulder press exercise lifting 20 pound dumbbells.

In today's workout you may set the challenge that if there's only one thing that you accomplish, it's getting to 10 reps with those 20 pound dumbbells.

Now, you have a mission. You've set something that you want to achieve in the gym that day and hopefully you'll be putting in the effort to make it happen. You have a *purpose* for going in there.

That's really all you want out of this – a *purpose*. When you feel as though you have a direct reason to hit the gym, you will. When you feel as though you don't have a reason – just that longer term goal looming ahead of you, that's when you won't.

So start setting those daily challenges. It can be whatever you want it to be as long as it's causing you to push yourself. That's the main thing here.

Include Plenty Of Variety In Cardio Activities

One of the big reasons why many people do experience boredom with their workout program and for good reason is because they simply are not doing enough variety when it comes to their activities.

Who can blame someone for getting bored when all they do is go into the gym day after day and hop on that treadmill? Not only are you bored, but you're not moving closer to your *end result* either as we've already illustrated numerous times over in this book.

What you need instead is to change it up a bit. Try a new cardio activity. Challenge yourself more. Get some muscles working in your body that have never been utilized before.

If you do this, that's when you're not only going to see a much greater interest in completing your workout sessions but when you're also going to see ten times the results as well.

Remember, the body always responds best to constant change so if you want to see maximum progress, always ensure that you are changing something about your workout sessions.

This includes moderate cardio workouts that you do alone. There are so many different options here – running, uphill walking, cycling, rowing, using the elliptical, rollerblading, swimming, walking, and so on that there really should be no reason why you're continuously doing the same thing over and over again.

If you are, you're literally asking for boredom to take place.

Some people may choose to change it up each and every workout – one day they're doing a jog and the next they're going for a bike ride, while others may choose to change it up on a week to week frequency.

Whatever you prefer, the key thing is that you're changing your workouts around frequently enough that you're preventing that boredom beast from creeping up.

When you do that, that's when you're on to results.

Workout At A Time When You Enjoy It

Finally, the last thing that you should be doing in effort to help maintain your motivational levels at an all time high is to make sure that you're working out at a time when you're actually going to enjoy it.

Some people do get stuck in the notion that a certain time is 'better' to exercise than others.

Sure, there are some specific advantage points to exercise at 'better times'. Such as people who do morning workouts tend to skip out on them less frequently and stick to their plan over the long haul as well as many people find they are stronger mid-afternoon when their body temperature is higher and they're full awake. This still does not discount the fact that in order for you to see any benefits whatsoever from your workout program you actually have to *do your workout program*.

Now how's that reasoning for you? While physiologically speaking there are a few select reasons for timing your workouts in a certain way, if you hate morning workouts with a passion and never get out of bed to get them in, they aren't really doing you a whole heck of a lot of good.

Instead, workout at a time when you're really going to enjoy it. When you're enjoying your workout and feeling your best you're going to put in that much more effort and as a result, the progress will be that much better.

Those who aren't enjoying their workouts will literally be sitting there counting down the minutes and this is in no way conducive to you seeing great results.

Workout enjoyment – both the time you choose to workout as well as the activities you're choosing to do is the single biggest determinant of your overall workout success.

Make no mistake about it, if you want to get results, you cannot be missing out on this point.

That now wraps up everything that you must be doing to stay motivated to stick with your workout program. Obviously you should also be taking the time to come up with your own unique strategies that work for you.

Perhaps you create a ritual where you always stop off for a massage at your last workout of the week provided all were completed or you make it a standing date to meet a friend for coffee on the way back from the gym (a calorie-conscious coffee, of course) – whatever the case, the important thing is that you learn what works for you.

What motivates one person to maintain their diet definitely does not always work for the next so making sure you figure out what's going to do it for you will be key.

Now we're going to move on to our next topic to cover as far as your workout success is concerned – alcohol. Many people do have numerous questions about whether or not they will be able to maintain their drinking habits as they go about their workouts and this will make things clearer for you.

CHAPTER 33:
ALCOHOL AND YOUR NEW LIFESTYLE

Friday night hits and your friends invite you out for a night on the town. Or, perhaps you're not going out with your friends but rather are spending a relaxing night in with your significant other and want something to help you wind down after a hard week and set the mood.

Whatever the case, for many people alcohol serves to be part of their regular lifestyle.

But at what cost?

That's what you really have to ask yourself if you're looking to get the absolute best results from your workout program. In many cases it really does boil down to just how intensely you want to see optimal results.

If you're someone who won't settle for anything less than getting absolutely everything you can from your workout program and dietary efforts, then alcohol is likely something you really should not be including in your day.

If you're alright with getting good results but are also willing to sacrifice slightly so that you can enjoy a drink now and then, then obviously your approach is going to change.

The one thing that you should be doing though is taking the time to learn how alcohol will influence your results so then you can make sound judgements based on that for what you should be doing.

Here are a few of the key things that you must remember at all times.

Alcohol and Calorie Intake

The very first thing that must be taken into consideration and quite possibly the most important aspect with regards to drinking alcohol and your progress is the calorie intake that you'll be facing from your drinking.

Depending on what your drink of choice is, this will have a very large influence over just how many calories you consume. Keep in mind that it's very possible for some of those fancier cocktails to get up to around 500-600 calories total once all the mixers and added ingredients go into the blender.

Have just three or four of those over the course of your evening and you could have very well cancelled out all the calorie deficit progress you made over the entire week!

They may taste delicious but when you place them alongside almost any dessert that you could have instead, it puts it into perspective just how many calories you're taking in.

A slice of cheesecake or a fancy cocktail?

Both often contain the equivalent number of calories. And, you know just how guilty you often feel from 'cheating' on your diet with a piece of cheesecake if it wasn't in fact a planned cheat (where there should be no guilt), so you have to ask why people are so willing to down these beverages without so much as a second thought?

The actual alcohol itself contains seven calories per gram so it rates in there right between carbs/protein and dietary fat which have four and nine respectively.

This makes it more calorie dense than if you were to have a plate of pasta and a chicken (gram for gram) so that factor will put you at an increased risk of fat gain.

Typically though it isn't even the alcohol calories itself that are the biggest problem – it's the mixers that go with it.

You add alcohol to either sugar or high-fat cream (if you're drinking liquors or creamy beverages) and then that's when you see the big problems developing.

Some drinks will also mix two variations of alcohol along with the mixers, again upping the overall calorie count and making it that much more detrimental to your weight loss progress.

If you are really dead set on including alcohol in your diet, it's a very wise move to try and avoid all these mixers if at all possible.

Also, avoid creamy liquors as they contain fat and alcohol calories – a powerful combination for distributing body fat right where you don't want it – your hips and thighs.

Instead, if you absolutely must drink, go with a regular lighter alcohol such as vodka and drink it with either water or diet soda (still not optional due to all the artificial ingredients).

This will come in at about 70-80 calories per ounce of alcohol so will not add up nearly as quickly. If you drink four or five over the course of the night that will still be 400-500 calories but at least you're not getting that in a single drink like you would with some of the other options!

So right off the bat, considering the calorie intake you take in from alcoholic beverages is the first issue to address. If you aren't aware of this and just drink at your leisure without cutting back on your calorie intake from other areas that day, it will set you back.

But *still*, cutting back on healthy foods to make room for alcohol is an extremely big problem and a very unwise thing to do (which is a big reason you see so many malnourished alcoholics out there – they drink rather than eat properly) so that really shouldn't ever be an option either.

Potentially the only thing you could cut out if you know you will be indulging in a few drinks that evening would be some of your starchy carbs from the diet. Since these aren't providing as many vital nutrients to the body as your lean protein sources are as well as the vegetables you're taking in, if one area of your diet must be cut back, this is where it should be.

Never, never, never cut back on your protein intake. Protein is a <u>must</u> for maintaining lean body mass and you must reach your target each and every day.

Alcohol and The Fat Burning Process

Second, the next big problem that you need to keep in the back of your mind with alcohol is that as soon as you take one drink, fat burning is essentially going to stop immediately.

You could be well on your way making progress with your workouts and burning off body fat faster than ever but the moment that alcohol enters your system fat burning gets shut off entirely.

This is due to the fact that the body has a certain hierarchy that it needs to follow that works in order of importance. Since alcohol is essentially considered a toxin to the body – something that will harm it and puts it in danger, when alcohol is present in the system, the absolute first priority is getting it removed.

It hits the liver and the body starts working hard to clear it from the blood stream and get the body back to its original state. In all of the effort, fat burning, an incredibly non-essential task gets pushed to the wayside.

As you go about your fat loss diet, when you take in that alcohol drink, you put the brakes on your progress. You're only going to pick back up on fat loss once all the alcohol has been cleared of the system and the energy from the drinks you took in (which often contain glucose – the body's preferred source of fuel) has been used up.

Drink enough alcohol and you could be looking at quite some time before you're back in the game of fat loss again.

You have to ask yourself, is it really worth it?

Alcohol and Will-Power

Now we move on to the next issue with regards to alcohol and one that most of you know all too well – alcohol can completely destroy your will-power.

You may have the best of intensions on your diet and are dead set on sticking with your program every second of the way but once you get a few drinks in you, all of a sudden that piece of chocolate cake is way too good to pass up.

Or, perhaps you figure that nothing would taste better with your beer than a nice plate of spicy chicken wings.

Sound familiar?

Now, not only are you taking in all the calories from the alcohol but you're also taking in all the calories from the food you consume. And typically, when you're drinking, the foods you consume are salty hence you eat a little bit and just want *more*.

Again, this dramatically ups your overall calorie intake and will pack on fat faster than ever.

Going back to the whole process of fat loss stopping as soon as alcohol enters the system, when you have all this food coming in now you not only have to clear the alcohol from your body but you must burn off a good 500-1000 calories along with it.

Now are you starting to see why drinking can be such a problem?

Sure, if you just go in and have one or two vodka's with water or diet Coke you aren't going to do too much damage, but go in and have four or five beers or two to three Margarita's along with some nachos and some pie to finish off the night and you're definitely looking at some serious problems as far as your weight loss progress goes.

Alcohol and Recovery Rates

In addition to all of the calorie issues that you're going to run into when consuming alcohol, the next problem you face is with regards to drinking and your workout progress.

You don't need me to tell you that if you go out drinking Friday night and enjoy yourself quite thoroughly that there's a very high chance that you won't be making your early Saturday morning workout sessions.

This is a given unless you are someone who is either able to push through a massive hangover or someone who just doesn't get hung-over in the first place.

So right away, missed workout sessions are obviously your first concern. If you're drinking too often and it's causing you to miss out on workouts that you should be doing, that will significantly decrease the overall rate of results that you see.

Second though, and possibly more important is the issue that alcohol ingestion will have on your recovery rates.

Once again, since alcohol is considered to be a toxin the body, when you ingest it the body no longer places recovery from your workout sessions as the priority.

And since you should know by now that immediately after a workout – for those first few hours especially, is 'prime' recovery time and after that it slows down significantly, you should clearly be able to see now why drinking can hinder you.

If you do a workout immediately after work and then come home and have a few drinks, you're really shorting the recovery that takes place.

This means that those muscles will not be built up as they should be and that you won't be able to give full effort next time you're in the gym. This means less intense workouts and fewer over all results for you.

Again, alcohol hinders your progress.

Alcohol and Muscle Building

Finally, the last big issue with alcohol is the issue of alcohol and muscle building. If you are someone who isn't as concerned with fat loss and thinks that this means they have the green light to have a drink whenever they want, you may want to reconsider.

Even though you may not be entirely concerned with the calorie intake from the alcohol or that it turns off fat burning (since for you, you aren't in a process of fat burning since your body is actually building up muscle tissue), you still must be very concerned with the overall recovery rate issue.

If you're working hard in the gym you're tearing down your muscle tissues each and every workout and if you don't give the muscles enough time to recover properly after that, when you hit the gym next time you're just going to be moving backwards in progress rather than forwards.

Drinking alcohol can actually set you back in your recovery up to two days total so it's not like it's just going to hinder you for a few hours either.

If you train on a Thursday evening and go out and get very intoxicated Friday night, you may not get the most of any sessions you do over the weekend.

Even worse would be training Friday morning and then drinking heavily Friday evening – you're really going to set yourself back by doing so.

There's all the information you must remember when thinking about alcohol intake and your progress.

It's fairly unrealistic to assume that most people will forgo drinking altogether. Like eating, it does have a social element to it and for many people, it is something they enjoy just as much, if not more, than eating some of their favorite 'cheat' foods.

They actually often bring up the question – for my 'cheat' meal, can I just go out drinking?

If this is something you're wondering, again, you must weigh the pros and cons. Sure, you may consume a similar amount of calories with a night drinking as you would with a full cheat meal or day however, with the cheat meal or day you're actually putting nutrients in the body that it can *use*.

There is a difference. The body actually has zero function for alcohol calories while with the cheat meal, you're still going to get *some* protein for muscle repair and more than likely plenty of carbohydrates which can get shuttled into the glycogen-depleted muscles and help you see faster recovery and even increase your metabolism (when done properly).

As you can see there is a difference. Sure, you can use alcohol as a cheat meal if you'd really like but you're not going to get quite the same benefits as you would if you hadn't.

Now let's move on and talk about another lifestyle factor that you must be aware about and make sure that you are considering in your program plan – sleep.

If you want to get results, you can't miss out on this.

CHAPTER 34:
SLEEP AND FAT LOSS

Sleep; Now there's something that almost every single person reading this book right now probably wishes they could get more of. Getting in your regular workouts is enough of a challenge with your busy schedule, getting in more sleep?

Now that's laughable!

But, if you really want to see better results, it's time to start making sleep a priority.

I know, ...'if only you could add another two hours to your day'.... And so the story goes. Making time for sleep is very difficult when you have a very busy lifestyle but if you want to truly succeed at weight loss, it's something that must be done.

Remember too that when you are well rested you're much more productive during the day so this will in fact almost make it seem as though you have found those few extra hours in the day as well.

But getting back to sleep and your progress, let's take a quick look at why sleep is vital for success.

Increased Hunger Levels

Ever had a very restless night the evening before – or just didn't get to bed until the wee hours of the morning and had to be up at 6 am to get to work and found that your stomach felt like a bottomless pit?

If so, you aren't alone. When you're running on low sleep it's far more likely that hunger is going to be a huge obstacle for you in your fat loss diet.

When you don't sleep enough, your body is going to send off these signals and increase your desire to eat and more often than not, since you are tired, it's sending these signals for carb-rich foods.

This explains why you may get much greater food cravings on days you're tired – your body is seeking a quick-energy source to turn to and it really needs to look no further than to that bagel, croissant, box of crackers, or piece of cake.

All are simple carbs that will cause an instant spike in your blood glucose level and instantly deliver you more energy.

Since on a fat loss diet your goal is to regulate your calories and take in fewer than the body would ideally like, this is going to make your day miserable.

Decreased Recovery

Second, the next big problem with lack of sleep is that sleep is the body's main time to recover from all your workout sessions.

If you're not sleeping on a daily basis, you aren't recovering either. If the situation is bad enough that could actually mean you start losing lean muscle mass rather than maintaining it or even building it.

Translation? A lower overall metabolic rate meaning you are less likely to continue to lose body fat into the future.

Ideally you should be getting seven to eight hours per night – eight is much better, to give the body the time it needs to repair those torn muscle tissues and make sure they are built back strong enough so that you're fully ready during your next workout.

Higher Levels Of Cortisol

Third, one particular hormone in the body – cortisol, is a hormone that's going to be released in much higher concentrations when you're low on sleep.

Cortisol is also your enemy. Why is it something that must be avoided?

Cortisol is going to encourage muscle mass breakdown so you move further away from that toned, firm body you're after and more importantly, it's also going to encourage body fat accumulation in the stomach region.

Obviously this is precisely what you don't want so minimizing cortisol will be essential. Stress brings on high levels of cortisol as does lack of sleep.

Increased Stress Eating

Another big issue that most people will find they deal with when low on sleep is that they're that much more tempted to eat when stressed out.

Everything just seems *that* much more overwhelming when you're incredibly tired because you just don't have the reserves you want to deal with it.

You're tired, you want to sleep, and the last thing you want to be doing is dealing with problems.

When you're stressed and tired, that will definitely spell trouble. Rather than dealing with it in the calm and collective manner you otherwise may have, you turn to food for comfort.

You're stressed and the only thing that's going to help you right this instant is that chocolate brownie you saw in the fridge.

Hence you eat it, trying anything possible to deal with your situation.

Temporarily you may actually feel better, but that brownie isn't going to solve the problems and once the blood sugar crash hits a short while after eating it, you'll be back for more – with a vengeance.

If you frequently fall into the trap of stress eating while running on low sleep, this will most definitely influence your results.

Reduced Glucose Tolerance

Finally, the last issue with low sleep is that it will also limit your body's ability to deal with incoming carbohydrates as well. Many people do find that they notice sharper blood sugar rises and crashes after eating a higher carbohydrate snack or meal when they are running low on sleep so this could also prompt you to eat more food, taking in more calories than you should.

In an ideal world, when you eat a carbohydrate rich food your body would take that glucose that gets broken down and shuttle it off right into the muscle cells.

But when you're low on sleep, this is often not what happens. Instead, the glucose will sit there in the blood stream giving you a temporary 'high' feeling before you crash, leaving you irritable, hungry, and at an all time low.

When you have enough sleep each night, your body will be better able to deal with the food you're feeding it and use it in the precise manner it should.

So as you can see, getting enough sleep is really vital to your overall success. Many people underestimate just how much low amounts of sleep can influence their results and in some cases, getting to bed earlier may even be *more* beneficial than you pushing through that hard workout session.

As crazy as it sounds, if you're incredibly tired you would be better off staying home and going to sleep than getting that workout in. You're not going to be able to put in nearly the same amount of effort anyway since you are so tired so there really is no advantage to doing so.

Sleep – aim for seven to eight hours per night and you will see the difference in your overall results.

Now we'll move on to our final topic to cover in the lifestyle section of this book that I do want to touch upon – stress. I already mentioned this briefly numerous times so far but this section will be specifically devoted to it.

CHAPTER 35:
TAKING CONTROL OF STRESS

When speaking of stress, it's important to realize that there are two main kinds of stress. You have positive stress and then you have negative stress.

Positive stress is going to enhance your life. It's going to serve to help energize you and motivate you to move forward and work towards your goals.

This stress serves to keep you at a higher level of awareness as you go about your day so you're better able to put forth all the effort you require to complete tasks that are needed.

Negative stress though – this is the stress that literally *eats away at your system*.

Not only does it cause the body to break down the tissues due to the fact that it's releasing that hormone called cortisol, but it also is going to put you at risk for a number of diseases as well.

If you really want to avoid long-term health complications, avoiding this stress will be a must.

What are some of the best coping techniques to help you manage your stress?

Let's look at the options (and these are just suggestions based on what works best for others):

- Get lost in your favorite book. For most people, reading and eating don't go together nearly as well as eating and watching TV do, so this is a far better way to spend your leisure time. Pick up a good book and as you get immersed, you may find you hardly even think about the food any longer.

- Go to a good comedy or thriller movie that makes you forget your worries. Often, getting out of the house is the fastest way to beat a food craving so don't overestimate the benefits of doing so. See a movie with a friend instead and pick up a pack of gum if you have to in order to avoid the concession stands.

- Call a friend and vent –sometimes simply 'getting it out there' helps relieve you of whatever it is that's stressing you. For anyone out there who tends to deal with emotional eating, sometimes the best way to stop yourself is to talk about what it is that's bothering you. Remember, food is only a cover up to the problem – it will still be there when you're finished your meal or snack and then you'll also have those added calories to deal with as well. Call a friend for advice instead.

- Write in a journal – in some cases, you'll feel more comfortable getting these thoughts out in private. If you aren't quite comfortable with the above suggestion, consider using a journal instead. Some people prefer to keep things private but even the act of writing it down on paper can help you release the emotions that are causing you to eat.

- Take a long hot bath to ease any tension build-up in the body. If you find that you eat because of stress and tension, rather than adding to your problems and creating more stress, do something that will reduce it. Take a hot bath and relax. This will improve your mood instantly and often you'll find when you get out, your craving has completely vanished.

- Come up with a 'thankful for' list – write down everything that has or is going well in your life so you don't just dwell on the stressors. This can really help put things in perspective and is another great way to cure emotional eating.

- Think about your 'worst case scenario' and what you'll do to get out of it – very often we figure the 'worst case scenario' is actually far worse than it really is. This exercise will bring that to awareness and help you realize that whatever it was that you were worried about just isn't all that bad.

- Speak to a counsellor – sometimes you just have to get professional help. Counsellors can often show you special tools and techniques that you can use to manage your stress and emotional eating tendencies that you just wouldn't get from talking with a friend.

- Do something for someone else – giving back can be just the cure for battling stressful times. By placing the focus on someone else for a change rather than yourself, you may temporarily forget whatever was troubling you and prevent overeating from taking place.

- Practice saying 'no'. If time is what's stressing you out, it's time to start putting a priority on your mental well-being and not taking on more than you can handle.

So there you have just a few ideas to get you started. Remember that what kills stress for you may not for someone else, so make sure that you're coming up with your own solutions.

It's also incredibly important that you're working to reduce whatever it is that is stressing you out in the first place.

Far too often we take a 'fix-it' stance as far as stress is concerned and rather than actually coming up with a viable solution to stop the stress initially, we just learn to mask it with our stress-reducing techniques.

While this can still prove to be somewhat beneficial as there are some things in life where you simply just cannot reduce the stressor, in other cases there are.

Perhaps it's a friend in your life who's always asking you to do things for him or her and you simply just do not have the time. If this is what's causing you stress, it's something that is easy to take care of.

First, speak to them about the behaviour and the stress it's causing you.

If they still don't understand, then it will be time to start practicing saying no. If they are a true friend, they should understand the situation and stop making any requests that simply are unnecessary or not reasonable.

By assessing your own individual situation and determining what it is exactly that is stressing you out you can come to better terms with whether or not it's going to be something you can deal with and manage.

If it is, take steps towards reducing it so it's not a factor in your life any longer. If it isn't, then you'll have to turn to your coping methods to get you through.

That now brings us to a close on your total transformation program. If you've read and fully understood this book, you are well on your way to getting your *end result*.

Even better, if you take action now and make sure to come see us in the studio, then we're going to be customizing each and every detail that we've already discussed to be sure that it's specific for you.

Remember that this is a very key and integral part of this equation. If you want to see the utmost success, you should be doing everything possible to tailoring it to your own individual body.

In the last section you'll find below I've included a number of helpful tools and resources for you to utilize to make your journey that much more comfortable.

You'll find recipes to try out with your diet plan as well as all the exercise descriptions from the workout program to ensure that you're completing everything correctly.

Always be careful that you are using proper form as it is going to be <u>vital</u> to preventing injuries, getting results from your workout plan, and making sure that you enjoy the entire process of this transformation.

CONCLUSION

So there you have everything that you need to know to get started on your journey to realizing your *end result*. It may feel slightly overwhelming at first trying to navigate through everything and find the path that works for you, which is why joining up with End Result Fitness is such a wise move.

When you train with us, we're going to be there every step of the way. You won't have to feel confused any longer about the best approach to take to realize your goals but instead will have a clear understanding of precisely what you should do to find success.

Whether you want to lose fat, firm up the body, improve your one mile running time, or gain functional strength that will help you as you go about your everyday life, you can be assured that we will reach those goals together.

End Result

FITNESS

YOUR 14 DAY KICK START PROGRAM
Success Journal

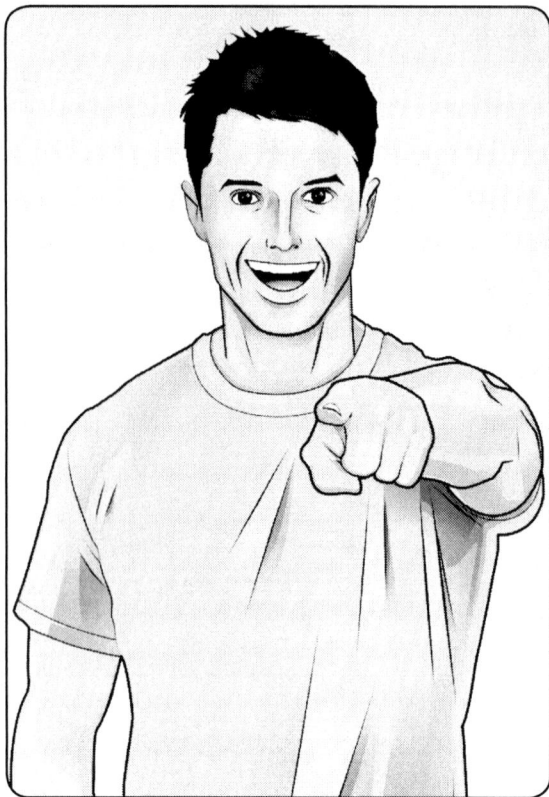

Welcome to the End Result Fitness family.

I am so happy and excited to be sharing this new program with you!

I feel very confident that this new program will help you set goals, kick ass and improve your quality of life.

You are just a few quick steps away from achieving your goals and becoming our very next **SUCCESS STORY!**

Let's take that first step today! No procrastinating. No concern with perfection. Just a few small steps today that lead to a giant leap tomorrow.

With the **14 Day Kick Start Program** you will eat more often. You'll learn how to lose fat to reshape your body into an even sexier shape. You'll also learn how to build lean, toned muscle tissue to increase your metabolism. This is all possible without completely giving up the foods you love. Your plan will consist of eating lean proteins, complex carbs, and healthy fats. These practices will keep your blood-sugar levels stable to help you stay satisfied and burn calories more efficiently.

The **14 Day Kick Start Program** will keep you lean, toned and healthy for the rest of your long life. This is not a fad diet; its a way of life that guarantees results!

We recommend the **14 Day Kick Start Program** at the beginning because it's easy to follow, it's better than what most people are doing right now, and it produces QUICK results in about 95% of our clients.

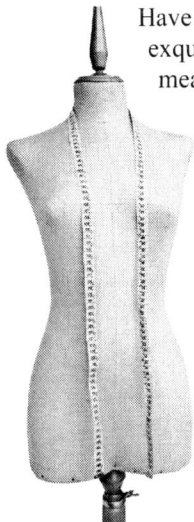

Have you ever watched a master tailor build a perfect, exquisitely tailored suit? From the stitching, to the repeated measurements and fittings, to the painstaking attention to detail, it's clear that making a custom suit is a complex process. But how does the perfect suit begin? It begins as a single, simple template. He begins with a template that's pretty general and then, with repeated tweaking, he modifies the suit for a better fit.

Your **14 Day Kick Start Program** follows a similar path: What begins as a broad template becomes a tailor-made nutrition plan through repeated measurements and adjustments.

Before we get started, please answer this very important question:

ARE YOU READY TO SET GOALS AND GET INTO THE BEST SHAPE OF YOUR LIFE?

❏ **YES!** I'm ready to set goals and get into the best shape of my life!

❏ NO! I'm not happy with the way I am, but I'm determined to stay that way.

If you answered "**YES!**" to the question above, congratulations! You've taken the first step toward achieving **YOUR** End Result. Now, let's get started!

allan alguire

V isualization is an important element for success in achieving your goals. Please attach a picture of yourself being at your goal weight (if you have that picture) on page 234. If you don't have one, then please attach a picture from a magazine of a person that has a similar body type and looks the way you want to look (your picture would be best though). Above your picture, is where you will also write down what I call your "Wish List". This is a very important "exercise" to complete before you actually begin your End Result Fitness workouts and nutrition program.

Please tap into your imagination and write down positive affirmations of all hopes, wishes, and dreams that come to mind when you think about successfully completing **YOUR** End Result Fitness Program; such as, "I love how confident I am", "I am less stressed at work", "I feel like I'm in my 20's again", "I have endless amounts of energy", "I love my life", etc. This reinforces what you desire and will quickly spark positive emotions, while we create a healthy, energetic, new you! Another reason this exercise is so powerful is that by bringing your subconscious health and fitness wishes to the surface, you'll be able to create very meaningful goals that are unique to you.

For more power, add images from magazines that provide you a visual of your positive affirmations you want to attract in your life as a result of completing **YOUR** End Result Fitness Program. Cut out the images and paste them to the page directly beside where you wrote down your "Wish List" (double-sided tape works best). There's no right or wrong way to do this exercise. Don't "over think" it - just do it. When you visualize them actually happening, you'll feel more energy, and **YOUR** End Result will happen quicker than you expect.

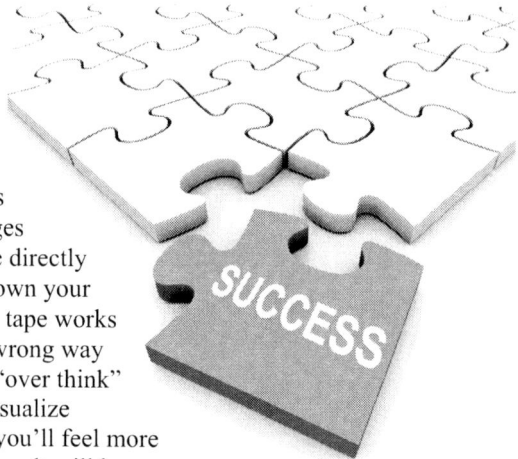

It's very important to understand the difference between wishes and goals. Wishes are things you dream for - things you enjoy thinking about but don't really know when or if they'll ever happen. Goals, on the other hand, are specific things you have committed to achieving within a clearly defined period of time. For example, "Someday I'm going to lose weight and get into shape" is a wish. "Over the next 12 months, I will lose 52 lbs of fat and get into the best shape of my life" is a kick ass goal. Notice that goals can be measured which will allow you and I to know that you've achieved them.

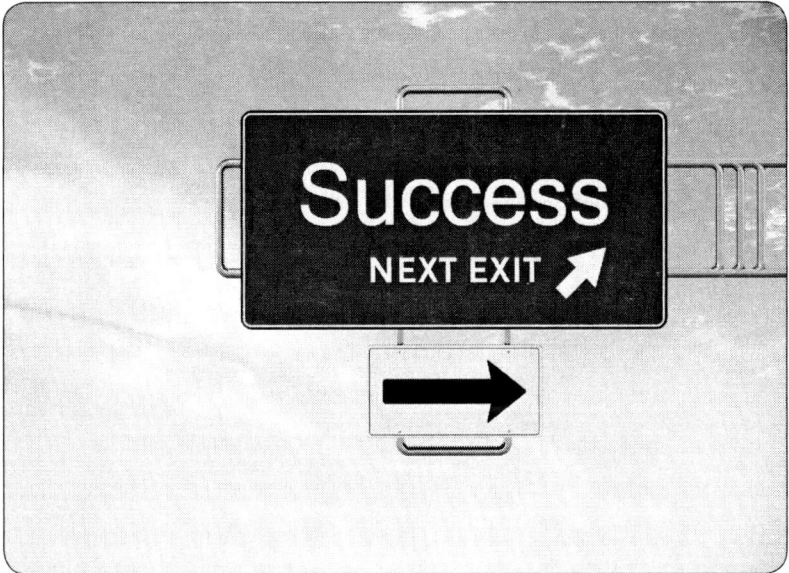

After you finish your Wish List, read it over again and let it serve as the inspiration for creating **YOUR** End Result Fitness goals.

Please write down positive affirmations of all hopes, wishes, and dreams that come to mind when you think about successfully completing **YOUR** End Result Fitness Program.

Attach picture here

End Result
F I T N E S S

Please add images from magazines that provide you a visual of your positive affirmations you want to attract in your life as a result of completing **YOUR** End Result Fitness Program.

MY KICK ASS GOALS:
Please write down 3 specific goals you will achieve over the course of your program. *Goals should be Specific, Measurable, Attainable, Realistic and Timely. In other words, in the goal setting process make sure you use the **SMART** system. You develop your goals from your Wish List. Once you clarify your goals, be sure to read them first thing in the morning and again at night.*

1

2

3

REASONS:
Please write down 3 reasons why you have decided to achieve your goals. *What I've discovered is that the more clear you are about why those goals are important to you, the more likely it is you'll succeed. It's not complicated at all to identify reasons for making changes to improve your health and fitness. There are countless reasons for wanting to become healthier, stronger, and more energetic. Be sure to write down three that have meaning to you. And please read your reasons every time you review your goals.*

1

2

3

REWARDS:
Please write down how you will reward yourself once you achieve your goals.

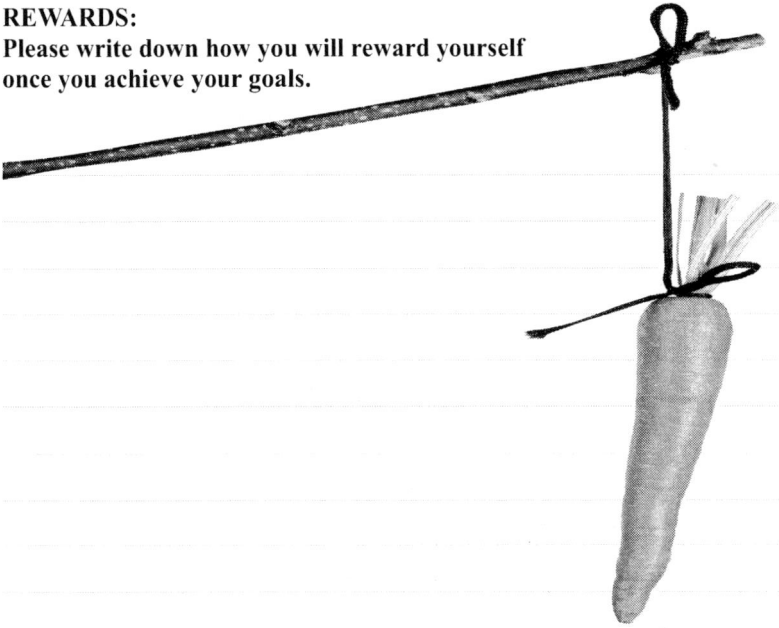

PUNISHMENT:
Please write down how you will punish yourself if you *give up* on achieving your goals.

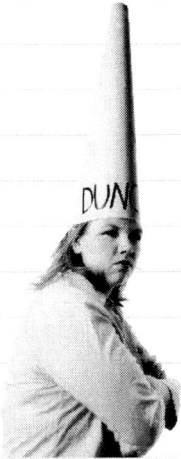

❏ Not applicable! I will not give up on achieving my goals. They are that important to me.

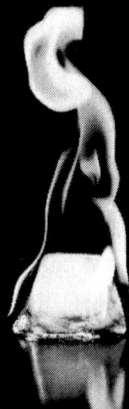

We've listed the **TOP** fat melting tips below. They're pretty straight forward - no PHD required. Although they may look simple, they're the product of years of research, testing them, experimenting with them, and modifying them until we had a system that could improve your body composition, health, energy levels and would guarantee your results if used faithfully. They also explain the three most important principles of any successful nutrition program. These are: When to eat, What to eat and how much to eat.

Tip #1 *Eat every 2-4 hours, and NO skipping meals*
Read those words again. When was the last time someone told you that you would lose weight by eating more? Answer: never!
Research has proven that eating every 2-4 hours is one of the most important strategies to improving health and body composition. Frequent eating (of well-chosen, properly sized meals and snacks) stimulates the metabolism, balances blood sugar, and helps maintain your LBM (Lean Body Mass) while giving your body a reason to burn off your extra stored energy, **FAT**.

Tip #2 *Count portion size not calories*
There aren't many people who can keep track of their calorie intake for an extended period of time. As an alternative, I recommend counting "portions". A proper portion of Lean Protein (L/P) is measured by what can fit in the palm of one hand. A proper portion of Complex Carbs from Fruit (FCC) and Vegetables (VCC) is measured by what can fit into two cupped hands and only one cupped hand for Starchy Complex Carbs (SCC). For Healthy Fats (H/F) a proper portion size would be one to two table spoons of healthy oil or one small handful of nuts.

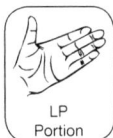

LP
Portion

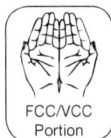

FCC/VCC
Portion

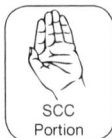

SCC
Portion

Tip #3 *Eat Lean Protein with every meal*
Lean Protein is the most integral part of muscle development. Since one pound of muscle burns approximately 50 calories a day, we want to ensure you are consuming enough protein to sculpt your lean, toned muscles in order to increase your metabolism. Also, Lean Protein takes more calories to breakdown in comparison to carbohydrates and fats. Every 100 calories of Lean Protein you eat will require 30 calories for breakdown and digestion. Now that's awesome.

Tip #4 *Eat Complex Carbs with every meal*
Try eating the majority of your Complex Carbs from fruits and vegetables (FCC, VCC). They are the best for getting lean. Plus they make you feel full without providing many calories. Vegetables and fruits also provide an alkaline load to the blood. Since both Lean Protein and Starchy Complex Carbs present acid loads to the blood, it's important to balance these acids with alkaline-rich, cancer fighting, free-radical destroying, and micro nutrient rich fruits and vegetables. Try eating Starchy Complex Carbs (SCC) with breakfast for long term energy throughout your day and 1-2 hours after exercise to replenish muscle glycogen but **ONLY** after your 14 Day Kick Start Program has ended. You've got to earn those Starchy Complex Carbs. When it comes to body composition change, sticking primarily with Complex Carbs from fruits and vegetables for the majority of your meals has been the single most effective strategy I've ever used to kick-start fat loss in clients with stubborn and hard to lose body fat stores.

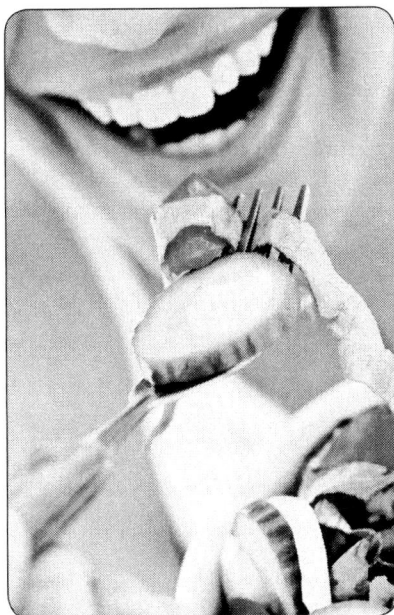

Tip #5 *Eat enough Healthly Fats*
Fat is a molecule of energy that can either be rapidly metabolized or stored. Some fat is required for optimal health, body composition and energy levels. Many doctors speak of the importance of omega - 3 fats, which the brain depends upon. Yes, in order to lose fat, get lean and keep the body looking great, you must eat fat. Even though "Good Fats" are good for you they still provide 9 kcal/gram, so please watch your portion sizes. Fat type is also important. Make sure your fat intake is balanced between

saturated, monounsaturated and polyunsaturated fat. I know you we're taught to fear saturated fats, but when saturated fat intake is balanced with a healthy amount of monounsaturated and polyunsaturated fat, you don't have to be afraid of it. Eating this way is easier than it looks. Just focus on adding the healthy monounsaturated fats (say, from extra virgin olive oil and avocado's) and polyunsaturated fat (say, from fish oil, flax seeds/oil, nuts and nut butters) into your diet. By ensuring you eat Lean Protein and Complex Carbs in every meal your dietary fat intake should balance itself right out.

Tip #6 *Don't drink beverages with more than 0 calories*
Eliminate fruit juice, soda, coffees and teas that are full of cream and sugar, plus any other sugary beverages from your diet. Drink water as your habitual beverage. Green tea, Herbal tea, Coffee, diet soda, Crystal light, in moderation, works too. Beyond these, stick with water for the most part. Protein shakes and or meal replacement shakes do not count as beverages, they are considered food. Since your body is made up of roughly 75% water and water is absolutely essential for a variety of physiological functions, your health, energy levels, and your body composition will suffer if you don't drink enough water. Make water part of every meal and it will soon become habit and you will never have to worry about not getting enough. When you drink cold water your metabolic rate is increased by as much as 30%. This happens because your body has to work harder to increase the temperature of the water to match that of your body.

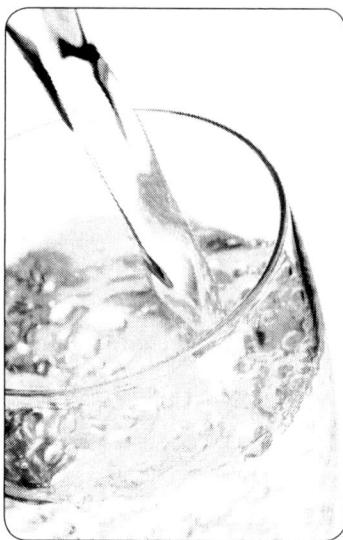

Also, lean muscle tissue is predominantly water. When muscles cells are full of water they help the muscle look toned and increase the body's ability to burn FAT. Try to drink about 12 cups, or a minimum of three litres, each day.

Tip #7 *Eat whole foods instead of supplements whenever possible*
Your food intake should come from high quality, largely unprocessed whole food sources. Sure, it's easier to grab an energy bar, a handful of mixed nuts or a protein shake than to prepare a whole food meal. However, it's best to get as many whole food meals as possible. Eat bars and shakes only when you're crunched for time or during the exercise/post exercise period when only liquid nutrition will do. No pills can even come close to matching the

vitamins and minerals that good old fruits and veggies contain. Don't rely on multivitamins; instead, eat a complete diet full of lean proteins, fruits and veggies, high fibre and nutrient dense starchy complex carbs (at the right times), and good healthy fats.

Tip #8 *Plan ahead and prepare food in advance*
The hardest part about eating well isn't necessarily understanding which foods are good and which are bad. Nor is it understanding proteins, complex carbs, and fats, or when to eat certain foods. The hardest part is consistency. Sometimes good nutrition is less about the food and more about making sure the food is available when it's time to eat. It's easy enough to eat well at home since you can stock your refrigerator, cupboards and pantry with wholesome, nutritious foods. However, as soon as you leave the house it becomes a far more difficult task. Can you trust what is in that salad you purchased around the corner from your office? Thus, you'll need to come up with food preparation strategies in order to ensure that you can consistently get the nutrition you need when you need it. Whether that means cooking a bunch of meals on Sunday for the upcoming week; getting up 30 minutes earlier and preparing food for the rest of the day; or hiring a food preparation service to do it for you, it's critical to have a plan. Remember! You will be as successful as you plan to be!

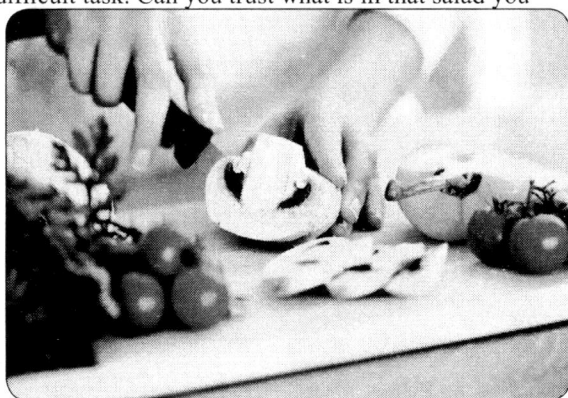

Tip #9 *Plan to break the rules 10% of the time*

There is no pressure to be perfect. In fact, my years of experience has taught me that unless you're getting ready to stand on a bodybuilding, fitness, or figure stage in a small posing outfit, the difference between 90% and 100% adherence is negligible. Also, from a psychological perspective, it's important to eat some food that don't necessarily follow the rules from time to time. So rather than expecting 100% adherence, we suggest 90% compliance. and that means you get to break the rules 10% of the time. Use the 10% meals as a source of pleasure, not stress. Schedule your 10% meals and enjoy them. (Don't pig out, though. Eating meals that are 3-4 times the size of your normal meals isn't the way to your goals and you know that already!) Pick a Saturday night meal, or a Sunday brunch, and eat some foods you wouldn't normally eat. Then, with your next meal, get back to your nutrition plan.

Tip #10 *NO breaking the rules for the first 21 days*
Please don't cheat on your nutrition plan for 21 days. It takes the brain 21 days to reset itself and create a new habit. When you want to make a change, don't tell yourself you are doing it for life; instead tell yourself you are going to try it for 21 days. Now, when you have completed this for 21 days, your conscious mind has the choice of stopping it or carrying on, or so it thinks. Your neural pathways have formed already and you will more than likely continue with your new habit. You will have seen and felt the benefits along the way and your subconscious mind will want to continue because it has been so beneficial.

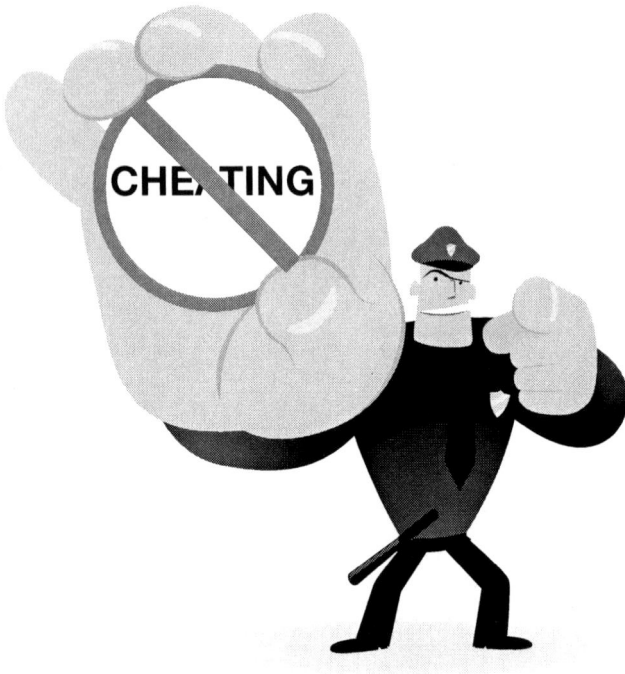

Lean Proteins (LP):

- Buffalo / Bison
- Venison
- Lean Ground Turkey
- Protein supplements
(milk protein, whey protein isolates, hemp protein, soy protein or rice protein)
- Fish
(Shrimp, Swordfish, Ahi Tuna, Halibut, Tilapia, Salmon, Cod, Mahi Mahi, Shark Steak, Red Snapper)
- Sushi / sashimi
- Canned tuna, packed in water
(low sodium)
- Egg Whites
(Simply Egg whites, Egg Creations)
- Omega-3 Eggs
- Boneless Skinless Chicken Breast
- Boneless Skinless Turkey Breast
- Pork Tenderloin

- Lean Red Meat
(93% lean, top round, flank, sirloin, extra lean ground beef, beef tenderloin)
- Turkey Bacon *(nitrate-free)*
- Low-Sodium Deli Meats
(turkey, ham, roast beef)
- Low Fat, Plain Yogurt
(lactose free if you can find it)
- Liberte Greek Yogurt, Plain 0% M/F
- Tofu
- Soy
(Veggie Burgers/Dogs/Ground, Sausage, Bacon)
- Tempeh
- Low-Fat Cottage Cheese
- Allegro 4% Milk Fat cheese
(preferably lactose free)
- Lactose Free Skim Milk

Starchy Complex Carbs (SCC):

Only after your 14 Day Kick Start Program has ended.

- Mixed Beans
(kidney, navy, pinto, soy) fat-free low-sodium*
- Quinoa*
- Whole Oats, Oatmeal
- Steel Cut Oats, Oatmeal
- Cream of wheat
- Rye Bread low-sodium
- All-Bran low-sodium cereal
- Kashi Go-Lean cereal
- Brown Rice
- Brown Rice cakes

- Couscous
- Ezekiel 4:9 bread, pasta, buns, English muffins and wraps
- Whole-grain pasta
(Eden Organic pasta company)
- Whole-grain wraps
- Sweet potatoes
- Yams
- Red potatoes
- Chickpeas*
- Lentils*
- Split peas*
- Bananas

*These are high-protein complex carbs and may be used as a protein source.
**Please refer back to FAT MELTING TIP #4

Vegetable Complex Carbs (VCC):

- Broccoli
- Green Beans
- Asparagus
- Brussels Sprouts
- Artichokes
- Cabbage
- Celery
- Cauliflower
- Carrots
- Cucumbers
- Eggplant
- Spinach
- Kale
- Lettuce
(except iceberg)
- Peas
- Onions
- Tomatoes
- Zucchini
- Mushrooms
- Peppers
(red, green, yellow)
- Pickles
- Bok Choy
- Pumpkin
- Turnip

Fruit Complex Carbs (FCC):

- Apples
- Berries
(blackberries, raspberries, blueberries, strawberries)
- Grapefruit
- Oranges
- Grapes
- Kiwi
- Pears
- Pomegranate
- Peaches
- Plums
- Pineapple
- Watermelon
- Mango
- Cherries

Healthy Fats (HF):

- Unsalted Almonds
- Avocados
- Walnuts
- Pine nuts
- Unsalted Pistachios
- Pecans
- Unsalted Cashews
- Nut Butters
- Cold - Water Fish
- Fish Oil Supplement
- Flaxseeds / oil
- Hazelnut Oil
- Extra Virgin Olive Oil
- Pumpkin seed Oil
- Pumpkin seeds
- Safflower Oil
- Sunflower seeds
- Virgin Coconut Oil
- Grated Unsweetened Coconut
- Udo's Oil
- Mazola Simplicity Extra Virgin Olive Oil No stick Cooking Spray

Condiments and Seasonings:

- Ketchup *(Blue Menu PC 65% Less Calories No Sugar Added)*
- Dijon Mustard
- Horseradish
- Cilantro
- Lite Tamari Soy Sauce *(low sodium)*
- Balsamic vinegar
- Tabasco
- Apple Sauce *(no sugar added)*
- Salsa *(no sugar added)*
- Lemon and lime juice
- Apple Cider Vinegar
- Sugar Twin
- Splenda
- Stevia
- Ginger
- Cinnamon
- Nutmeg
- Sage
- Thyme
- Rosemary
- Garlic
- Basil
- Oregano
- Black Pepper
- Tomato Sauce *(low sodium)*
- Sea Salt
- Onion
- Parsley
- Dill
- Cayenne
- Paprika
- Cumin
- Curry
- Dry Mustard

SAMPLE meal plan

Meal 1	Time 7:00 ☑ a.m. ☐ p.m.	**Meal 2**	Time 10:00 ☑ a.m. ☐ p.m.
LP: 2 eggs + 2 egg whites		LP: 1 scoop whey protein isolate	
SCC: ONLY AFTER 14 DAYS		SCC: ONLY AFTER 14 DAYS	
FCC: 1/2 cup Raspberries or Blueberries		FCC:	
VCC: 1/3 cup Red or Green Peppers		VCC: 8-10 mini-carrots (Raw)	
HF:		HF:	
H20: 2 cups water		H20: 2 cups water	
Other:		Other: 1 packlet of Crystal Light	
EXERCISE Time ____ ☐ YES ☑ NO		**EXERCISE** Time ____ ☐ YES ☑ NO	

Meal 3	Time 12:30 ☐ a.m. ☑ p.m.	**Meal 4**	Time 3:00 ☐ a.m. ☑ p.m.
LP: 1 grilled chicken breast		LP: 1 serving of any	
SCC: ONLY AFTER 14 DAYS		SCC: Quick and Easy	
FCC:		FCC: Anytime	
VCC: 1-2 cups steamed broccoli		VCC: SUPER	
HF: 1 tbsp Extra Virgin Olive Oil		HF: Shake or Bar	
H20: 2 cups water		H20: 2 cups water	
Other: 1 tsp of Sea Salt		Other:	
EXERCISE Time ____ ☐ YES ☑ NO		**EXERCISE** Time ____ ☐ YES ☑ NO	

Meal 5	Time 6:00 ☐ a.m. ☑ p.m.	**Meal 6**	Time 8:00 ☐ a.m. ☑ p.m.
LP: 1 grilled chicken breast		LP:	
SCC: ONLY AFTER 14 DAYS		SCC:	
FCC:		FCC:	
VCC: Steamed green beans		VCC:	
HF: 1 tbsp Extra Virgin Olive Oil		HF:	
H20: 2 cups water		H20:	
Other:		Other:	
EXERCISE Time ____ ☐ YES ☑ NO		**EXERCISE** Time ____ ☐ YES ☑ NO	

Appetite 0 1 2 3 4 5   **Sleep Quality** 0 1 2 3 4 5

Tiredness 0 1 2 3 4 5   **Willingness to train** 0 1 2 3 4 5

LEGEND

Appetite	Sleep Quality	Tiredness	Willing to train
0 = No Appetite	0 = Poor Sleep	0 = No Tiredness	0 = No willingness
5 = Very Hungry	5 = Very good sleep	5 = Very tired	5 = Very excited

LP = Lean Protein   **FCC** = Fruit Complex Carbs
HF = Healthy Fats   **SCC** = Starchy Complex Carbs
H2O = Water   **VCC** = Vegetable Complex Carbs

SAMPLE meal plan

Meal 1	Time 7:00 ☑ a.m. ☐ p.m.	Meal 2	Time 10:00 ☑ a.m. ☐ p.m.
LP: 1 cup Liberté Greek Yogurt, Plain 0% M/F		LP: 2 hard boiled Omega-3 Eggs	
SCC: ONLY AFTER 14 DAYS		SCC: ONLY AFTER 14 DAYS	
FCC: 1/2 cup Blueberries		FCC:	
VCC:		VCC: 3-4 Celery Sticks	
HF: 1 tbsp Almond Butter		HF:	
H2O: 2 cups water		H2O: 2 cups water	
Other: 1 Green Tea		Other:	
EXERCISE Time ___ ☐ YES ☑ NO		EXERCISE Time ___ ☐ YES ☑ NO	

Meal 3	Time 12:30 ☐ a.m. ☑ p.m.	Meal 4	Time 3:00 ☐ a.m. ☑ p.m.
LP: 1 small can Tuna drained (low sodium)		LP: 1 serving of any	
SCC: ONLY AFTER 14 DAYS		SCC: Quick and Easy	
FCC:		FCC: Anytime	
VCC: Dark green lettuce or spinach with veggies		VCC: SUPER	
HF: 1 tbsp Extra Virgin Olive Oil		HF: Shake or Bar	
H2O: 2 cups water		H2O: 2 cups water	
Other: Balsamic Vinegar		Other:	
EXERCISE Time ___ ☐ YES ☑ NO		EXERCISE Time ___ ☐ YES ☑ NO	

Meal 5	Time 6:00 ☐ a.m. ☑ p.m.	Meal 6	Time 8:00 ☐ a.m. ☑ p.m.
LP: 4 oz Salmon		LP:	
SCC: ONLY AFTER 14 DAYS		SCC:	
FCC:		FCC:	
VCC: 1-2 cups steamed Bok Choy		VCC:	
HF: 1 tbsp Extra Virgin Olive Oil		HF:	
H2O: 2 cups water		H2O:	
Other:		Other:	
EXERCISE Time ___ ☐ YES ☑ NO		EXERCISE Time ___ ☐ YES ☑ NO	

IF HUNGRY

Appetite 0 1 2 3 4 5 **Sleep Quality** 0 1 2 3 4 5

Tiredness 0 1 2 3 4 5 **Willingness to train** 0 1 2 3 4 5

LEGEND

Appetite	Sleep Quality	Tiredness	Willing to train
0 = No Appetite	0 = Poor Sleep	0 = No Tiredness	0 = No willingness
5 = Very Hungry	5 = Very good sleep	5 = Very tired	5 = Very excited

LP = Lean Protein **FCC** = Fruit Complex Carbs

HF = Healthy Fats **SCC** = Starchy Complex Carbs

H2O = Water **VCC** = Vegetable Complex Carbs

SAMPLE meal plan

Meal 1	Time 7:00 ☑ a.m. ☐ p.m.	**Meal 2**	Time 10:00 ☑ a.m. ☐ p.m.
LP: 4-6 Egg Whites		LP: 3/4 cup Librete Greek Yogurt, Plain 0% M/F	
SCC: ONLY AFTER 14 DAYS		SCC: ONLY AFTER 14 DAYS	
FCC: 1 medium apple		FCC: 1/3 cup Berries	
VCC:		VCC:	
HF:		HF:	
H20: 2 cups water		H20: 2 cups water	
Other:		Other: 1 packlet of Crystal Light	
EXERCISE Time____ ☐ YES ☑ NO		**EXERCISE** Time____ ☐ YES ☑ NO	

Meal 3	Time 12:30 ☐ a.m. ☑ p.m.	**Meal 4**	Time 3:00 ☐ a.m. ☑ p.m.
LP: 1 cup Lentils		LP: 1 serving of any	
SCC: ONLY AFTER 14 DAYS		SCC: Quick and Easy	
FCC:		FCC: Anytime	
VCC: 1-2 cups Vegetable Medley		VCC: SUPER	
HF: 1 tbsp Extra Virgin Olive Oil		HF: Shake or Bar	
H20: 2 cups water		H20: 2 cups water	
Other: Red Curry Spice		Other:	
EXERCISE Time____ ☐ YES ☑ NO		**EXERCISE** Time____ ☐ YES ☑ NO	

Meal 5	Time 6:00 ☐ a.m. ☑ p.m.	**Meal 6**	Time 8:00 ☐ a.m. ☑ p.m.
LP: 4 oz Beef Tenderlion		LP:	
SCC: ONLY AFTER 14 DAYS		SCC:	
FCC:		FCC:	
VCC: Grilled Asparagus		VCC: IF HUNGRY	
HF: 1 tbsp Extra Virgin Olive Oil		HF:	
H20: 2 cups water		H20:	
Other:		Other:	
EXERCISE Time____ ☐ YES ☑ NO		**EXERCISE** Time____ ☐ YES ☑ NO	

Appetite 0 1 2 3 4 5   **Sleep Quality** 0 1 2 3 4 5

Tiredness 0 1 2 3 4 5   **Willingness to train** 0 1 2 3 4 5

LEGEND

Appetite	Sleep Quality	Tiredness	Willing to train
0 = No Appetite	0 = Poor Sleep	0 = No Tiredness	0 = No willingness
5 = Very Hungry	5 = Very good sleep	5 = Very tired	5 = Very excited

LP = Lean Protein   **FCC** = Fruit Complex Carbs
HF = Healthy Fats   **SCC** = Starchy Complex Carbs
H2O = Water   **VCC** = Vegetable Complex Carbs

DAY 1 DATE: D/M/Y

Morning Resting Pulse   /BPM

Meal 1	Time ☐ a.m. ☐ p.m.	Meal 2	Time ☐ a.m. ☐ p.m.
LP:		LP:	
SCC:	ONLY AFTER 14 DAYS	SCC:	ONLY AFTER 14 DAYS
FCC:		FCC:	
VCC:		VCC:	
HF:		HF:	
H20:		H20:	
Other:		Other:	
EXERCISE	Time ☐ YES ☐ NO	**EXERCISE**	Time ☐ YES ☐ NO

Meal 3	Time ☐ a.m. ☐ p.m.	Meal 4	Time ☐ a.m. ☐ p.m.
LP:		LP:	
SCC:	ONLY AFTER 14 DAYS	SCC:	ONLY AFTER 14 DAYS
FCC:		FCC:	
VCC:		VCC:	
HF:		HF:	
H20:		H20:	
Other:		Other:	
EXERCISE	Time ☐ YES ☐ NO	**EXERCISE**	Time ☐ YES ☐ NO

Meal 5	Time ☐ a.m. ☐ p.m.	Meal 6	Time ☐ a.m. ☐ p.m.
LP:		LP:	
SCC:	ONLY AFTER 14 DAYS	SCC:	
FCC:		FCC:	
VCC:		VCC:	
HF:		HF:	IF HUNGRY
H20:		H20:	
Other:		Other:	
EXERCISE	Time ☐ YES ☐ NO	**EXERCISE**	Time ☐ YES ☐ NO

Appetite 0 1 2 3 4 5   **Sleep Quality** 0 1 2 3 4 5

Tiredness 0 1 2 3 4 5   **Willingness to train** 0 1 2 3 4 5

LEGEND

Appetite	Sleep Quality	Tiredness	Willing to train
0 = No Appetite	0 = Poor Sleep	0 = No Tiredness	0 = No willingness
5 = Very Hungry	5 = Very good sleep	5 = Very tired	5 = Very excited

LP = Lean Protein   **FCC** = Fruit Complex Carbs   **BPM** = Beats Per Minute

HF = Healthy Fats   **SCC** = Starchy Complex Carbs

H2O = Water   **VCC** = Vegetable Complex Carbs

DAY 2 **DATE:**

Meal 1	Time ___ ☐ a.m. ☐ p.m.	**Meal 2**	Time ___ ☐ a.m. ☐ p.m.
LP:		LP:	
SCC:	ONLY AFTER 14 DAYS	SCC:	ONLY AFTER 14 DAYS
FCC:		FCC:	
VCC:		VCC:	
HF:		HF:	
H20:		H20:	
Other:		Other:	
EXERCISE	Time ___ ☐ YES ☐ NO	**EXERCISE**	Time ___ ☐ YES ☐ NO

Meal 3	Time ___ ☐ a.m. ☐ p.m.	**Meal 4**	Time ___ ☐ a.m. ☐ p.m.
LP:		LP:	
SCC:	ONLY AFTER 14 DAYS	SCC:	ONLY AFTER 14 DAYS
FCC:		FCC:	
VCC:		VCC:	
HF:		HF:	
H20:		H20:	
Other:		Other:	
EXERCISE	Time ___ ☐ YES ☐ NO	**EXERCISE**	Time ___ ☐ YES ☐ NO

Meal 5	Time ___ ☐ a.m. ☐ p.m.	**Meal 6**	Time ___ ☐ a.m. ☐ p.m.
LP:		LP:	
SCC:	ONLY AFTER 14 DAYS	SCC:	
FCC:		FCC:	
VCC:		VCC:	IF HUNGRY
HF:		HF:	
H20:		H20:	
Other:		Other:	
EXERCISE	Time ___ ☐ YES ☐ NO	**EXERCISE**	Time ___ ☐ YES ☐ NO

Appetite 0 1 2 3 4 5 **Sleep Quality** 0 1 2 3 4 5

Tiredness 0 1 2 3 4 5 **Willingness to train** 0 1 2 3 4 5

LEGEND

Appetite	**Sleep Quality**	**Tiredness**	**Willing to train**
0 = No Appetite	0 = Poor Sleep	0 = No Tiredness	0 = No willingness
5 = Very Hungry	5 = Very good sleep	5 = Very tired	5 = Very excited

LP = Lean Protein **FCC** = Fruit Complex Carbs **BPM** = Beats Per
HF = Healthy Fats **SCC** = Starchy Complex Carbs Minute
H2O = Water **VCC** = Vegetable Complex Carbs

DAY 3   **DATE:** D / M / Y

Meal 1	Time ___ ☐ a.m. ☐ p.m.
LP:	
SCC:	ONLY AFTER 14 DAYS
FCC:	
VCC:	
HF:	
H20:	
Other:	
EXERCISE	Time ___ ☐ YES ☐ NO

Meal 2	Time ___ ☐ a.m. ☐ p.m.
LP:	
SCC:	ONLY AFTER 14 DAYS
FCC:	
VCC:	
HF:	
H20:	
Other:	
EXERCISE	Time ___ ☐ YES ☐ NO

Meal 3	Time ___ ☐ a.m. ☐ p.m.
LP:	
SCC:	ONLY AFTER 14 DAYS
FCC:	
VCC:	
HF:	
H20:	
Other:	
EXERCISE	Time ___ ☐ YES ☐ NO

Meal 4	Time ___ ☐ a.m. ☐ p.m.
LP:	
SCC:	ONLY AFTER 14 DAYS
FCC:	
VCC:	
HF:	
H20:	
Other:	
EXERCISE	Time ___ ☐ YES ☐ NO

Meal 5	Time ___ ☐ a.m. ☐ p.m.
LP:	
SCC:	ONLY AFTER 14 DAYS
FCC:	
VCC:	
HF:	
H20:	
Other:	
EXERCISE	Time ___ ☐ YES ☐ NO

Meal 6	Time ___ ☐ a.m. ☐ p.m.
LP:	
SCC:	
FCC:	
VCC:	IF HUNGRY
HF:	
H20:	
Other:	
EXERCISE	Time ___ ☐ YES ☐ NO

Appetite 0 1 2 3 4 5   **Sleep Quality** 0 1 2 3 4 5

Tiredness 0 1 2 3 4 5   **Willingness to train** 0 1 2 3 4 5

LEGEND

Appetite	Sleep Quality	Tiredness	Willing to train
0 = No Appetite	0 = Poor Sleep	0 = No Tiredness	0 = No willingness
5 = Very Hungry	5 = Very good sleep	5 = Very tired	5 = Very excited

LP = Lean Protein   **FCC** = Fruit Complex Carbs   **BPM** = Beats Per
HF = Healthy Fats   **SCC** = Starchy Complex Carbs   Minute
H2O = Water   **VCC** = Vegetable Complex Carbs

DAY 4 DATE: _D / M / Y_ *Morning Resting Pulse ___ /BPM*

Meal 1	Time____ ☐ a.m. ☐ p.m.	Meal 2	Time____ ☐ a.m. ☐ p.m.
LP:		LP:	
SCC:	ONLY AFTER 14 DAYS	SCC:	ONLY AFTER 14 DAYS
FCC:		FCC:	
VCC:		VCC:	
HF:		HF:	
H2O:		H2O:	
Other:		Other:	
EXERCISE	Time____ ☐ YES ☐ NO	**EXERCISE**	Time____ ☐ YES ☐ NO

Meal 3	Time____ ☐ a.m. ☐ p.m.	Meal 4	Time____ ☐ a.m. ☐ p.m.
LP:		LP:	
SCC:	ONLY AFTER 14 DAYS	SCC:	ONLY AFTER 14 DAYS
FCC:		FCC:	
VCC:		VCC:	
HF:		HF:	
H2O:		H2O:	
Other:		Other:	
EXERCISE	Time____ ☐ YES ☐ NO	**EXERCISE**	Time____ ☐ YES ☐ NO

Meal 5	Time____ ☐ a.m. ☐ p.m.	Meal 6	Time____ ☐ a.m. ☐ p.m.
LP:		LP:	
SCC:	ONLY AFTER 14 DAYS	SCC:	
FCC:		FCC:	
VCC:		VCC:	
HF:		HF:	IF HUNGRY
H2O:		H2O:	
Other:		Other:	
EXERCISE	Time____ ☐ YES ☐ NO	**EXERCISE**	Time____ ☐ YES ☐ NO

Appetite 0 1 2 3 4 5   **Sleep Quality** 0 1 2 3 4 5

Tiredness 0 1 2 3 4 5   **Willingness to train** 0 1 2 3 4 5

LEGEND

Appetite	Sleep Quality	Tiredness	Willing to train
0 = No Appetite	0 = Poor Sleep	0 = No Tiredness	0 = No willingness
5 = Very Hungry	5 = Very good sleep	5 = Very tired	5 = Very excited

LP = Lean Protein   **FCC** = Fruit Complex Carbs   **BPM** = Beats Per
HF = Healthy Fats   **SCC** = Starchy Complex Carbs   Minute
H2O = Water   **VCC** = Vegetable Complex Carbs

DAY 5　　　　　　　　**DATE:**　　　　　　　　Morning Resting
Pulse　　/BPM

Meal 1	Time　　　☐ a.m. ☐ p.m.	Meal 2	Time　　　☐ a.m. ☐ p.m.
LP:		LP:	
SCC:	ONLY AFTER 14 DAYS	SCC:	ONLY AFTER 14 DAYS
FCC:		FCC:	
VCC:		VCC:	
HF:		HF:	
H20:		H20:	
Other:		Other:	
EXERCISE	Time　　　☐ YES ☐ NO	**EXERCISE**	Time　　　☐ YES ☐ NO

Meal 3	Time　　　☐ a.m. ☐ p.m.	Meal 4	Time　　　☐ a.m. ☐ p.m.
LP:		LP:	
SCC:	ONLY AFTER 14 DAYS	SCC:	ONLY AFTER 14 DAYS
FCC:		FCC:	
VCC:		VCC:	
HF:		HF:	
H20:		H20:	
Other:		Other:	
EXERCISE	Time　　　☐ YES ☐ NO	**EXERCISE**	Time　　　☐ YES ☐ NO

Meal 5	Time　　　☐ a.m. ☐ p.m.	Meal 6	Time　　　☐ a.m. ☐ p.m.
LP:		LP:	
SCC:	ONLY AFTER 14 DAYS	SCC:	
FCC:		FCC:	
VCC:		VCC:	
HF:		HF:	
H20:		H20:	
Other:		Other:	
EXERCISE	Time　　　☐ YES ☐ NO	**EXERCISE**	Time　　　☐ YES ☐ NO

IF HUNGRY

Appetite 0 1 2 3 4 5　　　　**Sleep Quality** 0 1 2 3 4 5

Tiredness 0 1 2 3 4 5　　　　**Willingness to train** 0 1 2 3 4 5

Appetite	Sleep Quality	Tiredness	Willing to train
0 = No Appetite	0 = Poor Sleep	0 = No Tiredness	0 = No willingness
5 = Very Hungry	5 = Very good sleep	5 = Very tired	5 = Very excited

LP = Lean Protein	**FCC** = Fruit Complex Carbs	**BPM** = Beats Per
HF = Healthy Fats	**SCC** = Starchy Complex Carbs	Minute
H2O = Water	**VCC** = Vegetable Complex Carbs	

DAY 6   **DATE:**

Meal 1	Time___ ☐ a.m. ☐ p.m.	**Meal 2**	Time___ ☐ a.m. ☐ p.m.
LP:		LP:	
SCC:	ONLY AFTER 14 DAYS	SCC:	ONLY AFTER 14 DAYS
FCC:		FCC:	
VCC:		VCC:	
HF:		HF:	
H20:		H20:	
Other:		Other:	
EXERCISE	Time___ ☐ YES ☐ NO	**EXERCISE**	Time___ ☐ YES ☐ NO

Meal 3	Time___ ☐ a.m. ☐ p.m.	**Meal 4**	Time___ ☐ a.m. ☐ p.m.
LP:		LP:	
SCC:	ONLY AFTER 14 DAYS	SCC:	ONLY AFTER 14 DAYS
FCC:		FCC:	
VCC:		VCC:	
HF:		HF:	
H20:		H20:	
Other:		Other:	
EXERCISE	Time___ ☐ YES ☐ NO	**EXERCISE**	Time___ ☐ YES ☐ NO

Meal 5	Time___ ☐ a.m. ☐ p.m.	**Meal 6**	Time___ ☐ a.m. ☐ p.m.
LP:		LP:	
SCC:	ONLY AFTER 14 DAYS	SCC:	
FCC:		FCC:	
VCC:		VCC:	
HF:		HF:	IF HUNGRY
H20:		H20:	
Other:		Other:	
EXERCISE	Time___ ☐ YES ☐ NO	**EXERCISE**	Time___ ☐ YES ☐ NO

Appetite 0 1 2 3 4 5   **Sleep Quality** 0 1 2 3 4 5

Tiredness 0 1 2 3 4 5   **Willingness to train** 0 1 2 3 4 5

LEGEND

Appetite	Sleep Quality	Tiredness	Willing to train
0 = No Appetite	0 = Poor Sleep	0 = No Tiredness	0 = No willingness
5 = Very Hungry	5 = Very good sleep	5 = Very tired	5 = Very excited

LP = Lean Protein   **FCC** = Fruit Complex Carbs   **BPM** = Beats Per
HF = Healthy Fats   **SCC** = Starchy Complex Carbs   Minute
H2O = Water   **VCC** = Vegetable Complex Carbs

Meal 1	Time ____ ☐ a.m. ☐ p.m.	**Meal 2**	Time ____ ☐ a.m. ☐ p.m.
LP:		LP:	
SCC:	ONLY AFTER 14 DAYS	SCC:	ONLY AFTER 14 DAYS
FCC:		FCC:	
VCC:		VCC:	
HF:		HF:	
H2O:		H2O:	
Other:		Other: ·	
EXERCISE	Time ____ ☐ YES ☐ NO	**EXERCISE**	Time ____ ☐ YES ☐ NO

Meal 3	Time ____ ☐ a.m. ☐ p.m.	**Meal 4**	Time ____ ☐ a.m. ☐ p.m.
LP:		LP:	
SCC:	ONLY AFTER 14 DAYS	SCC:	ONLY AFTER 14 DAYS
FCC:		FCC:	
VCC:		VCC:	
HF:		HF:	
H2O:		H2O:	
Other:		Other:	
EXERCISE	Time ____ ☐ YES ☐ NO	**EXERCISE**	Time ____ ☐ YES ☐ NO

Meal 5	Time ____ ☐ a.m. ☐ p.m.	**Meal 6**	Time ____ ☐ a.m. ☐ p.m.
LP:		LP:	
SCC:	ONLY AFTER 14 DAYS	SCC:	
FCC:		FCC:	
VCC:		VCC:	
HF:		HF:	IF HUNGRY
H2O:		H2O:	
Other:		Other:	
EXERCISE	Time ____ ☐ YES ☐ NO	**EXERCISE**	Time ____ ☐ YES ☐ NO

Appetite 0 1 2 3 4 5   **Sleep Quality** 0 1 2 3 4 5

Tiredness 0 1 2 3 4 5   **Willingness to train** 0 1 2 3 4 5

LEGEND

Appetite	Sleep Quality	Tiredness	Willing to train
0 = No Appetite	0 = Poor Sleep	0 = No Tiredness	0 = No willingness
5 = Very Hungry	5 = Very good sleep	5 = Very tired	5 = Very excited

LP = Lean Protein   **FCC** = Fruit Complex Carbs   **BPM** = Beats Per
HF = Healthy Fats   **SCC** = Starchy Complex Carbs   Minute
H2O = Water   **VCC** = Vegetable Complex Carbs

DAY 8 DATE: _____

Meal 1	Time_____ ☐ a.m. ☐ p.m.	**Meal 2**	Time_____ ☐ a.m. ☐ p.m.
LP:		LP:	
SCC:	ONLY AFTER 14 DAYS	SCC:	ONLY AFTER 14 DAYS
FCC:		FCC:	
VCC:		VCC:	
HF:		HF:	
H20:		H20:	
Other:		Other:	
EXERCISE	Time_____ ☐ YES ☐ NO	**EXERCISE**	Time_____ ☐ YES ☐ NO

Meal 3	Time_____ ☐ a.m. ☐ p.m.	**Meal 4**	Time_____ ☐ a.m. ☐ p.m.
LP:		LP:	
SCC:	ONLY AFTER 14 DAYS	SCC:	ONLY AFTER 14 DAYS
FCC:		FCC:	
VCC:		VCC:	
HF:		HF:	
H20:		H20:	
Other:		Other:	
EXERCISE	Time_____ ☐ YES ☐ NO	**EXERCISE**	Time_____ ☐ YES ☐ NO

Meal 5	Time_____ ☐ a.m. ☐ p.m.	**Meal 6**	Time_____ ☐ a.m. ☐ p.m.
LP:		LP:	
SCC:	ONLY AFTER 14 DAYS	SCC:	IF HUNGRY
FCC:		FCC:	
VCC:		VCC:	
HF:		HF:	
H20:		H20:	
Other:		Other:	
EXERCISE	Time_____ ☐ YES ☐ NO	**EXERCISE**	Time_____ ☐ YES ☐ NO

Appetite 0 1 2 3 4 5   **Sleep Quality** 0 1 2 3 4 5

Tiredness 0 1 2 3 4 5   **Willingness to train** 0 1 2 3 4 5

LEGEND

Appetite	Sleep Quality	Tiredness	Willing to train
0 = No Appetite	0 = Poor Sleep	0 = No Tiredness	0 = No willingness
5 = Very Hungry	5 = Very good sleep	5 = Very tired	5 = Very excited

LP = Lean Protein   **FCC** = Fruit Complex Carbs   **BPM** = Beats Per
HF = Healthy Fats   **SCC** = Starchy Complex Carbs   Minute
H2O = Water   **VCC** = Vegetable Complex Carbs

DAY 9   **DATE:**   *Morning Resting*
                                                Pulse   /BPM

Meal 1	Time	☐ a.m. ☐ p.m.	Meal 2	Time	☐ a.m. ☐ p.m.
LP:			LP:		
SCC:	ONLY AFTER 14 DAYS		SCC:	ONLY AFTER 14 DAYS	
FCC:			FCC:		
VCC:			VCC:		
HF:			HF:		
H20:			H20:		
Other:			Other:		
EXERCISE	Time	☐ YES ☐ NO	**EXERCISE**	Time	☐ YES ☐ NO

Meal 3	Time	☐ a.m. ☐ p.m.	Meal 4	Time	☐ a.m. ☐ p.m.
LP:			LP:		
SCC:	ONLY AFTER 14 DAYS		SCC:	ONLY AFTER 14 DAYS	
FCC:			FCC:		
VCC:			VCC:		
HF:			HF:		
H20:			H20:		
Other:			Other:		
EXERCISE	Time	☐ YES ☐ NO	**EXERCISE**	Time	☐ YES ☐ NO

Meal 5	Time	☐ a.m. ☐ p.m.	Meal 6	Time	☐ a.m. ☐ p.m.
LP:			LP:		
SCC:	ONLY AFTER 14 DAYS		SCC:		
FCC:			FCC:		
VCC:			VCC:		
HF:			HF:		
H20:			H20:		
Other:			Other:		
EXERCISE	Time	☐ YES ☐ NO	**EXERCISE**	Time	☐ YES ☐ NO

IF HUNGRY

Appetite 0 1 2 3 4 5   **Sleep Quality** 0 1 2 3 4 5

Tiredness 0 1 2 3 4 5   **Willingness to train** 0 1 2 3 4 5

LEGEND

Appetite	**Sleep Quality**	**Tiredness**	**Willing to train**
0 = No Appetite	0 = Poor Sleep	0 = No Tiredness	0 = No willingness
5 = Very Hungry	5 = Very good sleep	5 = Very tired	5 = Very excited

LP = Lean Protein   **FCC** = Fruit Complex Carbs   **BPM** = Beats Per
HF = Healthy Fats   **SCC** = Starchy Complex Carbs   Minute
H2O = Water   **VCC** = Vegetable Complex Carbs

DAY 10 **DATE:**

Meal 1	Time___ ☐ a.m. ☐ p.m.	**Meal 2**	Time___ ☐ a.m. ☐ p.m.
LP:		LP:	
SCC:	ONLY AFTER 14 DAYS	SCC:	ONLY AFTER 14 DAYS
FCC:		FCC:	
VCC:		VCC:	
HF:		HF:	
H20:		H20:	
Other:		Other:	
EXERCISE	Time___ ☐ YES ☐ NO	**EXERCISE**	Time___ ☐ YES ☐ NO

Meal 3	Time___ ☐ a.m. ☐ p.m.	**Meal 4**	Time___ ☐ a.m. ☐ p.m.
LP:		LP:	
SCC:	ONLY AFTER 14 DAYS	SCC:	ONLY AFTER 14 DAYS
FCC:		FCC:	
VCC:		VCC:	
HF:		HF:	
H20:		H20:	
Other:		Other:	
EXERCISE	Time___ ☐ YES ☐ NO	**EXERCISE**	Time___ ☐ YES ☐ NO

Meal 5	Time___ ☐ a.m. ☐ p.m.	**Meal 6**	Time___ ☐ a.m. ☐ p.m.
LP:		LP:	
SCC:	ONLY AFTER 14 DAYS	SCC:	
FCC:		FCC:	
VCC:		VCC:	IF HUNGRY
HF:		HF:	
H20:		H20:	
Other:		Other:	
EXERCISE	Time___ ☐ YES ☐ NO	**EXERCISE**	Time___ ☐ YES ☐ NO

Appetite 0 1 2 3 4 5   **Sleep Quality** 0 1 2 3 4 5

Tiredness 0 1 2 3 4 5   **Willingness to train** 0 1 2 3 4 5

LEGEND

Appetite	Sleep Quality	Tiredness	Willing to train
0 = No Appetite	0 = Poor Sleep	0 = No Tiredness	0 = No willingness
5 = Very Hungry	5 = Very good sleep	5 = Very tired	5 = Very excited

LP = Lean Protein   **FCC** = Fruit Complex Carbs   **BPM** = Beats Per
HF = Healthy Fats   **SCC** = Starchy Complex Carbs   Minute
H2O = Water   **VCC** = Vegetable Complex Carbs

DAY 11   **DATE:** D / M / Y   *Morning Resting*
Pulse __ */BPM*

Meal 1	Time___ ☐ a.m. ☐ p.m.	Meal 2	Time___ ☐ a.m. ☐ p.m.
LP:		LP:	
SCC:	ONLY AFTER 14 DAYS	SCC:	ONLY AFTER 14 DAYS
FCC:		FCC:	
VCC:		VCC:	
HF:		HF:	
H20:		H20:	
Other:		Other:	
EXERCISE	Time___ ☐ YES ☐ NO	**EXERCISE**	Time___ ☐ YES ☐ NO

Meal 3	Time___ ☐ a.m. ☐ p.m.	Meal 4	Time___ ☐ a.m. ☐ p.m.
LP:		LP:	
SCC:	ONLY AFTER 14 DAYS	SCC:	ONLY AFTER 14 DAYS
FCC:		FCC:	
VCC:		VCC:	
HF:		HF:	
H20:		H20:	
Other:		Other:	
EXERCISE	Time___ ☐ YES ☐ NO	**EXERCISE**	Time___ ☐ YES ☐ NO

Meal 5	Time___ ☐ a.m. ☐ p.m.	Meal 6	Time___ ☐ a.m. ☐ p.m.
LP:		LP:	
SCC:	ONLY AFTER 14 DAYS	SCC:	
FCC:		FCC:	
VCC:		VCC:	IF HUNGRY
HF:		HF:	
H20:		H20:	
Other:		Other:	
EXERCISE	Time___ ☐ YES ☐ NO	**EXERCISE**	Time___ ☐ YES ☐ NO

Appetite 0 1 2 3 4 5   **Sleep Quality** 0 1 2 3 4 5

Tiredness 0 1 2 3 4 5   **Willingness to train** 0 1 2 3 4 5

LEGEND

Appetite	Sleep Quality	Tiredness	Willing to train
0 = No Appetite	0 = Poor Sleep	0 = No Tiredness	0 = No willingness
5 = Very Hungry	5 = Very good sleep	5 = Very tired	5 = Very excited

LP = Lean Protein   FCC = Fruit Complex Carbs   BPM = Beats Per
HF = Healthy Fats   SCC = Starchy Complex Carbs   Minute
H2O = Water   VCC = Vegetable Complex Carbs

DAY 12 **DATE:** _____ *Morning Resting*
Pulse */BPM*

Meal 1	Time _____ ☐ a.m. ☐ p.m.	Meal 2	Time _____ ☐ a.m. ☐ p.m.
LP:		LP:	
SCC:	ONLY AFTER 14 DAYS	SCC:	ONLY AFTER 14 DAYS
FCC:		FCC:	
VCC:		VCC:	
HF:		HF:	
H20:		H20:	
Other:		Other:	
EXERCISE	Time _____ ☐ YES ☐ NO	**EXERCISE**	Time _____ ☐ YES ☐ NO

Meal 3	Time _____ ☐ a.m. ☐ p.m.	Meal 4	Time _____ ☐ a.m. ☐ p.m.
LP:		LP:	
SCC:	ONLY AFTER 14 DAYS	SCC:	ONLY AFTER 14 DAYS
FCC:		FCC:	
VCC:		VCC:	
HF:		HF:	
H20:		H20:	
Other:		Other:	
EXERCISE	Time _____ ☐ YES ☐ NO	**EXERCISE**	Time _____ ☐ YES ☐ NO

Meal 5	Time _____ ☐ a.m. ☐ p.m.	Meal 6	Time _____ ☐ a.m. ☐ p.m.
LP:		LP:	
SCC:	ONLY AFTER 14 DAYS	SCC:	
FCC:		FCC:	
VCC:		VCC:	IF HUNGRY
HF:		HF:	
H20:		H20:	
Other:		Other:	
EXERCISE	Time _____ ☐ YES ☐ NO	**EXERCISE**	Time _____ ☐ YES ☐ NO

Appetite 0 1 2 3 4 5   **Sleep Quality** 0 1 2 3 4 5

Tiredness 0 1 2 3 4 5   **Willingness to train** 0 1 2 3 4 5

DAY 13   **DATE:** D / M / Y   *Morning Resting*
Pulse   /BPM

Meal 1	Time	☐ a.m. ☐ p.m.	**Meal 2**	Time	☐ a.m. ☐ p.m.
LP:			LP:		
SCC:	ONLY AFTER 14 DAYS		SCC:	ONLY AFTER 14 DAYS	
FCC:			FCC:		
VCC:			VCC:		
HF:			HF:		
H20:			H20:		
Other:			Other:		
EXERCISE	Time	☐ YES ☐ NO	**EXERCISE**	Time	☐ YES ☐ NO

Meal 3	Time	☐ a.m. ☐ p.m.	**Meal 4**	Time	☐ a.m. ☐ p.m.
LP:			LP:		
SCC:	ONLY AFTER 14 DAYS		SCC:	ONLY AFTER 14 DAYS	
FCC:			FCC:		
VCC:			VCC:		
HF:			HF:		
H20:			H20:		
Other:			Other:		
EXERCISE	Time	☐ YES ☐ NO	**EXERCISE**	Time	☐ YES ☐ NO

Meal 5	Time	☐ a.m. ☐ p.m.	**Meal 6**	Time	☐ a.m. ☐ p.m.
LP:			LP:		
SCC:	ONLY AFTER 14 DAYS		SCC:		
FCC:			FCC:		
VCC:			VCC:	IF HUNGRY	
HF:			HF:		
H20:			H20:		
Other:			Other:		
EXERCISE	Time	☐ YES ☐ NO	**EXERCISE**	Time	☐ YES ☐ NO

Appetite 0 1 2 3 4 5   **Sleep Quality** 0 1 2 3 4 5

Tiredness 0 1 2 3 4 5   **Willingness to train** 0 1 2 3 4 5

LEGEND

Appetite	**Sleep Quality**	**Tiredness**	**Willing to train**
0 = No Appetite	0 = Poor Sleep	0 = No Tiredness	0 = No willingness
5 = Very Hungry	5 = Very good sleep	5 = Very tired	5 = Very excited

LP = Lean Protein   **FCC** = Fruit Complex Carbs   **BPM** = Beats Per
HF = Healthy Fats   **SCC** = Starchy Complex Carbs   Minute
H2O = Water   **VCC** = Vegetable Complex Carbs

Meal 1	Time_____ ☐ a.m. ☐ p.m.	**Meal 2**	Time_____ ☐ a.m. ☐ p.m.
LP:		LP:	
SCC:	ONLY AFTER 14 DAYS	SCC:	ONLY AFTER 14 DAYS
FCC:		FCC:	
VCC:		VCC:	
HF:		HF:	
H20:		H20:	
Other:		Other:	
EXERCISE	Time_____ ☐ YES ☐ NO	**EXERCISE**	Time_____ ☐ YES ☐ NO

Meal 3	Time_____ ☐ a.m. ☐ p.m.	**Meal 4**	Time_____ ☐ a.m. ☐ p.m.
LP:		LP:	
SCC:	ONLY AFTER 14 DAYS	SCC:	ONLY AFTER 14 DAYS
FCC:		FCC:	
VCC:		VCC:	
HF:		HF:	
H20:		H20:	
Other:		Other:	
EXERCISE	Time_____ ☐ YES ☐ NO	**EXERCISE**	Time_____ ☐ YES ☐ NO

Meal 5	Time_____ ☐ a.m. ☐ p.m.	**Meal 6**	Time_____ ☐ a.m. ☐ p.m.
LP:		LP:	
SCC:	ONLY AFTER 14 DAYS	SCC:	
FCC:		FCC:	
VCC:		VCC:	IF HUNGRY
HF:		HF:	
H20:		H20:	
Other:		Other:	
EXERCISE	Time_____ ☐ YES ☐ NO	**EXERCISE**	Time_____ ☐ YES ☐ NO

Appetite 0 1 2 3 4 5   **Sleep Quality** 0 1 2 3 4 5

Tiredness 0 1 2 3 4 5   **Willingness to train** 0 1 2 3 4 5

YOUR PERSONAL TRAINERS COMMENTS

SHOPPING LIST

Lean Protein (LP)

❑ ....
❑ ....
❑ ....
❑ ....
❑ ....

Healthy Fats (HF)

❑ ....
❑ ....
❑ ....
❑ ....
❑ ....

Starchy Complex Carbs (SCC)

❑ ....
❑ ....
❑ ....
❑ ....
❑ ....

Fruit & Vegetable Complex Carbs
(FCC & VCC)

❑ ....
❑ ....
❑ ....
❑ ....
❑ ....

Quick And Easy SUPER Shakes and Bars

So what are **SUPER** shakes and bars? Well, for starters, Super Shakes and Bars are "meal replacements." The Super Shake and Bar are packed with good stuff like high-quality protein, fiber, good fats, antioxidants and more. The Super Shake and Bar aren't just a good meal replacement; it's actually superior to most of the meals your neighbors are eating all around you, all day long. In addition to the good nutrition it provides, the Super Shake and Bar meet your need for quick, easy, high-quality food that you can have in a pinch during your time-crunched schedule.

BREAKFAST or AFTER WORKOUT SUPER Shakes

Apple and Cinnamon Oatmeal SUPER Shake
(LP, SCC, FCC, VCC, HF)
1 cup water
1 scoop vanilla flavored whey protein isolate
1 serving greens supplement
1 tbsp ground flaxseeds
3 tbsp Liberte Greek Yogurt, Plain 0% M/F
4 tbsp whole grain oatmeal (dry)
1 tbsp natural almond butter
1 apple, peeled, corded and sliced
Cinnamon

Add water, protein, greens +, flax seed, yogurt and oats to a blender and blend on high for 1 minute. Next, add natural almond butter, apple slices and a sprinkle of cinnamon. Blend again for 1 minute. If you prefer an ice cold shake, add 5 ice cubes and blend for another minute.

**Makes 1 SUPER shake for men or
2 SUPER shakes for women.**

Berry Bliss Super Shake (LP, SCC, FCC, VCC)

1 cup iced green tea
1 scoop vanilla flavored whey protein isolate
1 serving greens supplement
3 tbsp Liberte Greek Yogurt, Plain 0% M/F
3 tbsp whole grain oatmeal (dry)
1 cup frozen or fresh mixed berries

Add green tea, protein, greens +, yogurt and oats to a blender and blend on high for 1 minute. Next, add berries to the blender and blend again for 1 minute.

Makes 1 SUPER shake for men or 2 SUPER shakes for women.

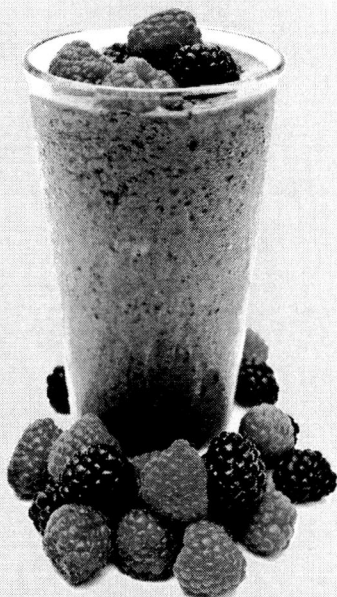

Strawberry and Banana SUPER Shake (LP, SCC, FCC)
1 medium banana
1 cup strawberries
1 cup lactose free skim milk
1 scoop strawberry whey protein isolate
1 cup ice
Splenda, to taste

Combine everything in a blender and process on medium-high until smooth and creamy. More ice may be added for a thicker texture.

Makes 1 SUPER shake for men or 2 SUPER shakes for women.

Veggie SUPER Shake (LP, VCC, HF)
1/4 cup parsley
1/2 cup spinach
3 carrots
2 celery stalks
1 glove garlic
1 scoop vanilla flavored whey protein isolate
1 serving greens supplement
1 tbsp ground flaxseeds

Place parsley, spinach, carrots, celery and garlic in a juicer. Dilute juice, if necessary, with cold water to achieve 1 cup of fluid. Add juice to blender along with protein, flax seeds and green +. Blend on high for 1 minute. If you prefer an ice cold shake, add 5 ice cubes and blend for another minute.

**Makes 1 SUPER shake for men or
2 SUPER shakes for women.**

Fruit and Veggie SUPER Special (LP, VCC, FCC, HF)
1 cup water
1 scoop vanilla flavored whey protein isolate
1 serving greens supplement
1/2 cup frozen or fresh blueberries
1/2 cup broccoli sprouts
1 raw beet
1 tbsp extra virgin olive oil
1/2 cup kale
1 cup ice

Add everything to blender and process until smooth and creamy.

**Makes 1 SUPER shake for men or
2 SUPER shakes for women.**

Yummy Turtle SUPER Shake (LF, VCC, HF)

1/2 cup water
1/2 cup ice cubes
2 scoops chocolate flavored whey protein isolate
1 tbsp greens supplement
1 oz chopped pecan halves
2 tbsp natural almond butter
1 cup egg whites

Add everything to blender and process until smooth and creamy.

**Makes 1 SUPER shake for men or
2 SUPER shakes for women.**

Almond Coconut SUPER Shake (LP, VCC, HF)

1 cup lactose free skim milk
1 scoop chocolate flavored whey protein isolate
1 serving greens supplement
1 tbsp natural almond butter
1 tbsp grated unsweetened coconut or virgin coconut oil
1 tbsp ground flaxseeds
1 cup ice

Add all ingredients to blender and process for one minute.

**Makes 1 SUPER shake for men or
2 SUPER shakes for women.**

Protein Coffee SUPER Shake (LP, VCC, HF)

2 cups iced coffee
2 scoops vanilla flavored whey protein isolate
1 serving greens supplement
Dash cinnamon
1 packet Sugar Twin or Splenda

Add everything to blender and process for 1 minute.

**Makes 1 SUPER shake for men or
2 SUPER shakes for women.**

Chocolate & Almond Bliss SUPER Shake (LP, VCC, HF)

1 cup water
1 scoop chocolate flavored whey protein isolate
1 serving greens supplement
3 tbsp Liberte Greek Yogurt, Plain 0% M/F
1 tbsp ground flaxseeds
1 tbsp natural almond butter

Add water, protein, greens +, yogurt and flaxseeds to blender and blend on high for 1 minute. Next add natural almond butter. Blend again for 1 minute. If you prefer an ice cold shake, add 5 ice cubes and blend for another minute.

**Makes 1 SUPER shake for men or
2 SUPER shakes for women.**

Tropical Power SUPER Shake (LP, VCC, FCC, HF)

1 cup water
1/2 cup Liberte Greek Yogurt, Plain 0% M/F
1/2 cup frozen or fresh pineapple
1 banana
1/4 cup of unsweetened coconut flakes or virgin coconut oil
1 scoop vanilla flavored whey protein isolate
1 tbsp greens supplement
1 tbsp grounded flaxseeds

Add everything to blender and process until smooth and creamy.

**Makes 1 SUPER shake for men or
2 SUPER shakes for women.**

Apple Cobbler Protein SUPER Bars (LP, SCC, FCC, HF)

1 cup oat flour
1 cup whole wheat flour
6 scoops strawberry or vanilla whey protein isolate
2/3 cup nonfat, plain, lactose free (if you can find it) yogurt
1 omega-3 egg
1 cup oat bran
1 cup granulated Splenda
1 cup applesauce, unsweetened
2 tbsp honey (with BeePolin if possible)
1 large apple, cored and chopped
2 tsp vanilla extract
2 tsp cinnamon
1/2 teaspoon sea salt
1 tbsp olive oil

Combine these in a large bowl: oat flour, whole wheat flour, sea salt, 2 tsp cinnamon, and most of the Splenda, leaving a couple of tablespoons for later. Stir these dry ingredients together. Put the yogurt, omega-3 egg, vanilla extract, and olive oil in a blender, and turn it on low. Add the whey protein isolate powder 1 scoop at a time, until thoroughly blended. Pour this mixture into the bowl, and stir together until it has the consistency of dough.

Coat a 9x13 inch baking pan with olive oil cooking spray, then pour the mixture into the pan, flattening it up to the edges. Next, mix the applesauce, 1 teaspoon cinnamon, chopped apples, and honey together, and pour over the top of the dough mixture in the pan, spreading evenly. Sprinkle the oat bran over the top, until thoroughly and evenly covered, and then sprinkle the remaining Splenda over the top. Bake for 15 minutes at 350-degrees F, and then switch to broil for 3-4 minutes, just until top is slightly browned. BE CAREFUL NOT TO OVERCOOK.

**Makes 12 SUPER bars for men or
15 SUPER bars for women.**

Cinnamon Raisin SUPER Bars (LP, SCC, FCC, HF)

2 cups large flake rolled oats
8 scoops vanilla whey protein isolate
1 cup raisins
1-1/2 cups unsweetened applesauce
1 tbsp olive oil or flax oil
2 tsp cinnamon
1 tsp sea salt
1 tsp vanilla extract
Splenda, to taste (about 1/2 cup granulated or 12-15 packets)

In a clean, dry blender, process one cup of rolled oats into flour (blend on medium for about 1 minute). Stir together the following ingredients in a large bowl: oat flour, the remaining rolled oats (1 cup), raisins, whey protein isolate powder, Splenda, cinnamon, sea salt. Stir the applesauce and vanilla extract together with the dry ingredients and mix thoroughly.

Cut 8-12 squares of aluminum foil, about 6x10 inches each. Lightly coat the interior with a olive oil cooking spray. Spoon out an equal portion of the mixture onto each foil square, and roll them into a bar shape. Fold them like tamales, folding the ends over to prevent spillage. You can flatten them into bar shapes if you want to avoid a tube-shaped bar.

Bake the bars in the foil in a preheated oven at 350-degrees F, for 16-20 minutes. BE SURE NOT TO OVERCOOK.

**Makes 6 SUPER bars for men or
10 SUPER bars for women.**

Mocha Espresso SUPER Bars (LP, SCC, HF)

1 cup oat flour
1 cup whole wheat flour
5 scoops chocolate whey protein isolate
1/2 cup whole espresso beans
1/2 tsp sea salt
Splenda, to taste (about 1 cup granulated)
1 omega-3 egg PLUS 1 egg-white, beaten
2 tbsp honey (with BeePolin if possible)
1 cup lactose free skim milk   *continued on next page*

Combine all of the dry ingredients in a large bowl, stir, and then add the eggs, honey and lactose free skim milk. Mix well, and then pour the dough into a 8x12 inch cooking dish. Bake at 350-degrees F for 12-15 minutes, or until a fork stuck into the center comes out dry. BE SURE NOT TO OVERCOOK OR IT WILL BECOME CHEWY AND TASTELESS.

**Makes 6 SUPER bars for men or
8 SUPER bars for women.**

Granola SUPER Bars (LP, SCC, FCC, HF)

2 cups large flake rolled oats
1/2 cup crushed walnuts
1/2 cup unpacked natural raisins (2 oz.)
4 tbsp whole flaxseeds
4 scoops vanilla whey protein isolate
2 tbsp honey (with BeePolin if possible)
1/4 tsp sea salt
1/4 tsp vanilla extract
1/2 cup sugar free maple syrup

In a large bowl combine the oats, walnuts, flaxseeds, raisins, and whey protein isolate. Add the honey, maple syrup, vanilla extract, and sea salt. Stir until everything is thoroughly mixed. At first, it will seem too dry, but continue stirring and it will eventually blend.

Coat a clean, dry 8x8 inch baking dish with olive oil cooking spray, then press the mixture into the bottom of the dish. The mixture should extend to all corners evenly, and it should be about 1-inch thick. You can also use a smaller baking dish for thicker, chewy bars. Bake at 350-degrees F for 10 minutes.

**Makes 8 SUPER bars for men or
12 SUPER bars for women**

Almond Butter Banana SUPER Bars (LP, SCC, FCC, HF)

8 scoops vanilla whey protein isolate
2 cups large flake rolled oats
4 medium bananas (Raw)
1.2 oz natural banana chips (about one handful)
4 tbsp chunky almond butter
1 cup granulated Splenda or 25-30 packets
1 tsp sea salt

In a clean, dry blender, process one cup of large flake rolled oats into flour (blend on medium for about 1 minute). After removing the oat flour, put the banana chips into the blender and chop into chips (only takes a few seconds). Put all of the dry ingredients into a large bowl and stir together: oat flour, the remaining rolled oats (1 cup), chopped banana chips, protein isolate powder, Splenda, Sea salt.

Slice the raw bananas into the blender and process on medium speed, until producing a puree. Add the almond butter and blend for a few seconds, just until mixed (you want to leave some almond chunks for texture). Stir the banana-almond butter puree together with the dry ingredients and mix thoroughly.

Cut 6-10 squares of aluminum foil, about 6x10 inches each. Lightly coat the interior with olive oil cooking spray. Spoon out on equal portion of the mixture onto each foil square, and roll them into a bar shape. Fold them like tamales, folding the ends over as well. You can flatten them into bar shapes if you want.

Bake the bars in the foil in a preheated oven at 350-degrees F, for 16-20 minutes. BE SURE NOT TO OVERCOOK.

**Makes 6 SUPER bars for men or
10 SUPER bars for women.**

Peanut Butter Fudge Bars (LP, HF)
4 scoops chocolate whey protein isolate
2/3 cup flax meal
4 tbsp chunky natural peanut butter
1/4 cup water
Splenda, to taste

Mix everything together in a large bowl and start stirring. At first, it will seem like it's not enough water, but keep stirring, and it will eventually become a sticky blob of dough. If you have to, add some water 1 tbsp at a time. Divide the mixture in 4-6 equal portions, and put them into separate pieces of plastic wrap, shaping into a bar within the wrap. It's easier to shape them by laying plastic wrap in one side of a small casserole dish, pressing the dough into a natural shape of the dish. Put the bars into the fridge, or store them in the freezer. You can eat them chilled, or even frozen, or you can eat it right out of the bowl if you're feeling impatient :)

Makes 4 SUPER bars for men or
6 SUPER bars for women.

Mixed Nut SUPER Bar (LP, HF)
3/4 cup pecan meal
3/4 cup almond meal
1/4 cup walnut pieces
2 whole omega-3 eggs
Plus 2 egg-whites, beaten
6 scoops vanilla whey protein isolate
1/4 tsp sea salt
Splenda, to taste (optional)

To make the pecan and almond meal, process the nuts in a blender. Mix everything together in a large bowl, and continue stirring until all of the ingredients have mixed together thoroughly. Spread the dough into an 8x8-inch backing dish coated with olive oil cooking spray and bake for 15 minutes at 350-degrees F.

Makes 6 SUPER bars for men or
10 SUPER bars for women.

Chocolate Almond Butter SUPER Bar (LP, HF)

1/2 cup pecan meal
1/2 cup almond meal
1/2 cup almond butter
1/3 cup flax meal
1 tbsp cocoa powder, unsweetened
1 whole omega-3 egg
Plus 1 egg-white beaten
6 scoops chocolate whey protein isolate
1/4 tsp sea salt
Splenda, to taste (about 6 packets or 1/4 cup of the granulated type)

Mix everything together in a large bowl. You will have to keep stirring to get everything to mix into a thick dough. Spread the mixture into a 8x8-inch baking dish coated with olive oil cooking spray. Bake for 12 minutes at 350-degrees F.

Makes 6 SUPER bars for men or
10 SUPER bars for women.

CARDIO INTENSITY LEVELS

Rate Of Perceived Exertion:

Use this scale to ensure that you're working out at the right intensity level for your Fat Blast and Calorie Torch Cardio sessions. Stay between level 4 and 6 for your Fat Blast sessions. For your Calorie Torch sessions stay at level 8 or 9 for your fast pace, and level 3 or 4 for your slow pace. Please also note that these speeds are merely guidelines. As you become fitter and your muscles get stronger, you'll naturally move faster and more efficiently at each of these levels.

LEVEL 1: Easiest. It's like I am sitting on the couch.

LEVEL 2: Easy. I could stay like this for a while.

LEVEL 3-4: Moderate. I am breathing harder, breaking a sweat, but I can still talk.

LEVEL 5: Moderately hard. I'm sweating, but I can still talk.

LEVEL 6-7: Hard. Okay, this is getting tough, I can talk in brief phrases, but rather not.

LEVEL 8: Insanely hard. I'm panting and grunting.

LEVEL 9-10: Too much! I can't keep this up.

FAT BLAST CARDIO - Steady-paced cardio sessions burn off fat. Do your cardio at a brisk pace (4-6 intensity level)

CALORIE TORCH CARDIO - Interval cardio sessions raise your metabolism and therefore calorie burn during and after your workout to shed even more fat. Alternate slower pace (3-4 intensity level) with short bursts of (8-9 intensity level)

YOUR EVALUATION

SKIN FOLDS / BODY COMPOSITION

DATE	D/M/Y	D/M/Y	D/M/Y	D/M/Y	D/M/Y	D/M/Y	D/M/Y	D/M/Y	D/M/Y	D/M/Y
Body Weight (lbs)										
Abdominal (mm)										
Tricep (mm)										
Subscapular (mm)										
Suprailiac (mm)										
Thigh (mm)										
Total of Skinfolds (mm)										
Body Fat %										
Fat Mass (lbs)										
LBM (lbs)										

MEASUREMENTS

DATE	D/M/Y	D/M/Y	D/M/Y	D/M/Y	D/M/Y	D/M/Y	D/M/Y	D/M/Y	D/M/Y	D/M/Y
Chest (inches)										
Waist (inches)										
Hips (inches)										
Right / Left Arm (inches)	R/L	R/L	R/L	R/L	R/L	R/L	R/L	R/L	R/L	R/L
Right / Left Thigh (inches)	R/L	R/L	R/L	R/L	R/L	R/L	R/L	R/L	R/L	R/L
Right / Left Calf (inches)	R/L	R/L	R/L	R/L	R/L	R/L	R/L	R/L	R/L	R/L